Broken Fragments

BROKEN
FRAGMENTS

Jewish Experiences
of Alzheimer's Disease
through Diagnosis, Adaptation,
and Moving On

Edited by Douglas J. Kohn

URJ Press • New York

For permission to reprint, please contact:

URJ Press
633 Third Avenue
New York, NY 10017-6778
212-650-4120
press@urj.org

Library of Congress Cataloging-in-Publication Data

Broken fragments : Jewish experiences of Alzheimer's disease through diagnosis, adaptation, and moving on / edited by Douglas J. Kohn.
   p. cm.
   Includes bibliographical references.
   ISBN 978-0-8074-1198-8
   1. Alzheimer's disease. 2. Dementia. 3. Alzheimer's disease—Patients—Care. 4. Alzheimer's disease—Patients—Biography. 5. Aging—Religious aspects—Judaism. 6. Aging parents—Care—Religious aspects—Judaism. 7. Memory—Religious aspects—Judaism. 8. Mental health—Religious aspects—Judaism. 9. Medicine—Religious aspects—Judaism. 10. Caring—Religious aspects—Judaism. 11. Caregivers—Religious life. 12. Spiritual life—Judaism. 13. Jewish ethics. I. Kohn, Douglas.
   RC523.2.B76 2012
   616.8'31—dc23
                                                                    2012011092

Printed on acid-free paper

Manufactured in the United States of America

10 9 8 7 6 5 4 3 2 1

To the memories of

my loving grandfather, David Kohn (z″l),
my patient father-in-law, Jack Bloom (z″l),
and our teacher and commentator, Rabbi W. Gunther Plaut (z″l),

each of whom surrendered their memories to Alzheimer's disease,
bequeathing yesterday and tomorrow to those of us who care,

and to every one in each of our families
whom dementia is touching,
as we remember that
every life is of
inestimable
worth

Contents

Part II • Adaptation

Part II • Moving On

Foreword

꩜

SIMKHA Y. WEINTRAUB

In truth, I was supposed to write a chapter for this book. The insightful and generous editor initially invited me to contribute, knowing that my family has been impacted by a loved one's dementia. In a struggle that lasted several months, I found myself feeling honored and privileged—but ultimately too challenged and overwhelmed—by this invitation. I declined, guilt-ridden and depleted by the inner grappling.

Why? Because—and this is the bottom line—the journey of a loved one's cognitive deterioration is truly beyond words. As the remarkable voices in this collection express, with penetrating honesty and astute self-observation, the degradation and loss, the chaos and despair, are without parallel. Alzheimer's disease and other causes or forms of dementia can take us to a precipice—repeatedly, sometimes hourly—of confusion and loneliness. We search for the person we know and love, for our own place and purpose, and for a measure of divine meaning or direction—something, somehow, somewhere.

And it's even worse than that. Just as one of the most important dimensions that distinguish human beings from fellow primates is language and social interaction, one of the features that have made Jews distinct from some other groups is our profound commitment— maybe obsessive at times—to memory. It seems that few things are more important for a Jew than to remember: the Creation, the Exodus, Shabbat—indeed, all the mitzvot—and from the experience of oppression in Egypt and the vile attacks of Amalek, to the centrality of Zion and Jerusalem. In our hearts and minds, proud admonitions such as "Remember where you came from" echo alongside more prosaic Jewish cautions such as "Remember what I told your brother when *he* went off to college . . ."

The microcosmic Jewish family reflects that macro. My family, like yours, is built on memories, articulated or implicit. When we gather for Shabbat or a seder or Thanksgiving, or anything else, stories—from the unspoken to the rehashed—are what bind and nurture us. And then a parent or a grandparent begins to lose his rudder, his vocabulary, before our very eyes. Before long, we are all at a loss and feel lost.

Remember, remember, remember; it is the key to identity, integrity, and sense of self and an essential component to finding one's way in life. Jewish behaving, believing, belonging, and just being seem to hinge on access to memory. "A scattered nation which remembers its Past and connects it with the Present, will undoubtedly have a Future as a people and probably even a more glorious life than the one in the Past," said the Russian Jewish journalist and fiction writer Lev Osipovich Levanda.[1] Or even more starkly, the Russian Jewish poet Elias Lieberman summarized, "Memories are all we really own."[2]

So what can we possibly do when the bottom begins to fall out, when the links have not only been disconnected but have disappeared, nowhere to be found?

On the High Holy Days, our liturgy borrows a line from Psalm 71: "Do not send me off at the season of old age; as my powers diminish, do not abandon me" (Psalm 71:9). That's a nice and compelling sentiment, to be sure, but it acquires special force as our *machzor*, our High Holy Day prayer book, recasts it in the plural form: "Do not send us off at the season of our old age; as our powers diminish, do not abandon us."

Hold that petition for a moment as I share with you one of the most powerful things I have heard in my twenty years of leading Jewish spiritual support groups through the New York Jewish Healing Center. At the conclusion of one meeting of a group for Jews living with life-altering chronic illnesses, one devoted and deeply spiritual member, Ellen Schecter, exclaimed, "You know what I love about this group? Our bodies are discreet—but our spirits overlap!" That is, our suffering is, alas, ours alone—nobody can truly feel our pain or fully plumb our desolation. Granted. But at least some relief and reassurance, and often lifesaving sustenance and even moments of unexpected transcendence, can derive from a community of honest, open fellow travelers. In the words of a popular Jewish folk saying, *Tzarat rabim chatzi nechamah*, "Sorrow shared is sorrow halved."

That is how this book truly sings. The contributors, a wide range of clergy and health professionals, form a protective circle of concern, attending to and sharing their own lived experience and hard-earned wisdom. Each in their own idiom and speaking from different vantage points on the journey, they draw on Jewish traditional sources as well as on the Torah of their lives, yielding a moving and helpful, but flexible and empowering framework for coping and hoping.

When all is said and done, our appeal—"Do not send us off at the season of our old age; as our powers diminish, do not abandon us"—is directed not only to the Almighty, but to the Jewish community, to society, to humanity. The concentric circles of patient, caregivers, family, and community require such enduring presence, support, and love. Because the only way one can navigate one's own chapter is in relation to others. I may yet begin to articulate my own.

Preface

❧

Douglas J. Kohn

The Talmud recalls that after Moses shattered the first set of Ten Commandments, destroying them with the Golden Calf, Moses did not discard those tablets' broken fragments. Although he returned to Mount Sinai to replace the tablets of the Ten Commandments, the shattered shards of the earlier set also were retained. "Respect the aged, because the fragments of the original tablets were preserved in the Ark with the new ones" (Babylonian Talmud, *B'rachot* 8b).

Alzheimer's disease represents a human set of *broken fragments*— of people and of memory. Just as the shattered pieces of the original tablets were broken due to no fault of their own—they were the victim of circumstance—so, too, those with Alzheimer's disease and other dementias are a human set of broken fragments due to no fault of their own. They, too, are subject to circumstance, a debilitating medical circumstance.

Memory is the currency of the Jew. It is the core command of the Erev Shabbat *Kiddush* prayer—to remember God's two great achievements of Creation and liberating the Jews from Egypt—and it is the cudgel of the aggrieved, lonely Jewish grandmother, demanding attention. It is the consistent, winnowing thread weaving through the weft of the Jewish people's four-millennia tapestry, recalling triumph and tragedy, and it is the foundation on which today's "Never again!" is voiced so viscerally in remembrance of our people's tragic, twentieth-century martyrdom. Memory is the intellectual and spiritual inheritance and privilege of each individual Jew, each of whom is endowed by God with the wondrous and mysterious gifts of mind, spirit, and body, which together capture, record, and archive not only historic events of eternal meaning, but also each of the modest, mundane episodes of a person's particular, individual life.

Thus, when memory is lost to an illness such as Alzheimer's disease or related dementia, the person suffers more than mere forgetfulness; she undergoes a compounding and cascading loss that purloins not only her personal narrative and story, but also her place in a family and her place in history. Moreover, along with the loss of memory itself, a person with Alzheimer's disease or dementia commonly also loses basic occupational abilities, such as dressing oneself, handling a phone, or using a fork, which, as fundamental skills, are silently but skillfully built on bodily, physiological memory. Thus, not only can the person no longer cognitively place himself in the events and sequences of his life, but also he no longer can participate effectively in those events. Finally, with these losses ultimately comes the strong possibility of losing dignity—the implanted, indwelling image of God—which situates the human being in God's glorious esteem in a privileged position "little lower than the angels."

If memory is the currency of the Jew, then how do Judaism, Jewish texts, and Jewish teachings help us to understand or cope with its loss? What can we learn from our tradition that may support or guide us to retain that precious divine esteem when it appears so vulnerable to vanishing? How do we evolve new systems and relationships to reflect the changing cognitive needs and abilities of dear ones with dementia? What ought we do, and what ought we refrain from doing, in order to be the best son or daughter, spouse or caregiver, to one with Alzheimer's disease? Ultimately, what is the Jew without memory, and what is our task, alongside him or her?

It has been said that Alzheimer's disease may be an epidemic. In the Western world, where health advances are resulting in significantly longer life spans than were expected just a generation ago, it may very well be true. Americans are aging and living ever longer, and with aging, the potential to be afflicted with Alzheimer's disease rises dramatically. Present data[1] indicate that while currently an estimated five and a half million people are living with Alzheimer's disease in America, 13 percent of those over age sixty-five are afflicted, while 43 percent of those over age eighty-five have the disease. Moreover, on average, Alzheimer's disease patients live from five to twenty years with their disease. Thus, it is evident that addressing, accommodating, and accepting Alzheimer's disease, as well as understanding it and its impact on both the person it afflicts and the person's family, are pressing contemporary concerns. As well, with the aging of America's baby boom generation, and as baby boomers retire and adjust to their own aging, experts are predicting a vast forthcoming increase in the incidence of Alzheimer's disease and related dementias. Today, there are nearly four hundred thousand new cases of Alzheimer's disease diagnosed annually; in thirty years, when the last of the baby boomers reach age sixty-five, the number of diagnoses is expected to have increased by 150 percent annually. And, with generally above-average fiscal resources that allow for access to medical care, those in the Jewish community are especially benefiting from health increases and longevity, and our numbers with Alzheimer's disease and dementia likely will exceed the norm. In addition to the heavy human toll, the financial costs due to Alzheimer's disease are staggering: the annual average cost of caregiving per family: $12,500; the average length of nursing home stay per patient: 2.5 years; the average cost of nursing home care per patient: $139,000; the annual cost of caregiver absenteeism to business: $7.89 billion; the annual cost of lost productivity due to work disruptions of caregivers: $26 billion; and the average annual cost to the U.S. economy: $100 billion.[2] Alzheimer's disease is a major concern for everyone.

Alzheimer's disease and dementia are not merely a collection of massive numbers; rather, they are faces and stories and people. Just after

I was ordained a rabbi in 1987, both my grandfather, David Kohn, and my father-in-law, Jack Bloom, were diagnosed with Alzheimer's disease. Though I briefly describe their stories in chapter 16, I would mention that the contrast between their rich, playful, able minds and souls in their higher, healthy years and their losses and regressions while with Alzheimer's disease is the glowing, orange firebrand that has seared the sorrow of Alzheimer's disease into my heart, and which in part inspires this book and this endeavor to offer Jewish meaning to the experience of Alzheimer's disease. Both David Kohn and Jack Bloom had great facility with numbers: my grandfather in studying the stock values in the daily newspaper, and Jack, a produce broker, every evening adding and collating lengthy lists of orders and figures from his clients—with pencil and paper. Both eventually became only broken fragments as their once-proficient minds degenerated, yet as the Talmud prescribes, their fragmented shards have been preserved in the arks of my family's lore and now help prompt the themes of this manuscript.

This volume, *Broken Fragments*, addresses a significant vacuum in the literature of Judaism, health, spirituality, and ethics and attempts to bring a measure of caring and hope to a concern that appears so very hopeless. Among all the wonderful books enriching the world of Jewish healing, the arena of Alzheimer's disease is unattended. Likely, this is both due to its painful difficulty and because thinkers just are not tackling the nexus of Jewish life and disease. Addressing Alzheimer's disease through a Jewish prism is a timely task.

Adding the Jewish perspective to our lens for viewing this disease offers the reader additional, vital tools with which to manage oneself and one's situation. The brilliance of our teachers—from the biblical writers to modern scholars—adds layers to the substrate on which we stand. Not only do we no longer stand alone in dealing with dementia, but we have the riches of our greatest minds who also have suffered and worried through such challenges and loss. Moreover, if our worldview or internal framework includes Judaism and its teachings and values, then we would naturally turn to our tradition for its wisdom and counsel when other views leave us wanting, helpless, and hopeless. It is hoped that by mining Judaism's textual gems, we might find some wisdom for the reader.

Admittedly, however, this is not an easy book to read. Unlike my earlier book addressing cancer and Judaism, the theme of this volume offers no prospect for a cure, nor even for a remission. As of this writing, as our physicians will tell us later, there is no potential on the viewable horizon for such a medical breakthrough. Thus, this book somewhat violates the traditional Jewish custom of offering a *nechemta*—a consolation. When a haftarah portion for a given Shabbat concludes with a pessimistic concluding verse, our Sages prescribed that an additional verse be added to the portion as a countervalance, so that the worshiper may depart positively, with hope.

What hope then, can this volume presume to offer when addressing Alzheimer's disease or dementia? Such is the spiritual challenge of writing this text: we sorely seek a fleeting or missing *nechemta*. Yet, there *are* consolations, and our writers will candidly and sensitively offer what they have discovered through working with those with Alzheimer's disease as clergy and physicians, as social workers and academics, as family members. We are reminded by their touching experiences and their compelling chapters that people with Alzheimer's disease are, indeed, still people, and we are reminded of rich and memorable moments that still may arise, even when a dear one has debilitating dementia. We are stirred to recall and reinvigorate our own humanity and our own sensitivity and gentleness, especially when we look again into that unique stare of one whose eyes once twinkled so sweetly and knowingly and we realize that their simple, daily value comes from our most patient expressions of love. We learn from our tradition, which teaches that we are "not to stand idly by another's blood" (Leviticus 19:16), that instead we are charged to stand—or sit—and make the day brighter alongside another who has this disease. We learn to find the *nechemta* in the simplest, most raw moments—but that is where they are to be found.

This book originated in one such moment. In a passing telephone conversation with my rabbinic friend and colleague Rabbi Andrew R. Sklarz of Greenwich, Connecticut, who later would contribute a wonderful chapter to this volume, the idea of the book was germinated. In 2009, Rabbi Sklarz was struggling with his mother's dementia and was seeking Jewish insights so he could meld his Jewish framework and his filial obligations into one consistent refinement. On the telephone that day, Rabbi Sklarz urged that a book comparable to my earlier cancer volume was needed now to address Judaism and Alzheimer's disease. His suggestion prompted this project, and I extend to him my gratitude for his inspiration and imagination.

As much as this book is not easy to read, it has not been easy to prepare. Finding Judaic texts that teach about dementia has been challenging. Jewish writings only tangentially or perhaps metaphorically address the phenomenon of age-related cognitive impairment, such as Alzheimer's disease. It has required careful and imaginative reading of our sacred texts in order to distill such meaning. As well, identifying the proper contributors for this volume was similarly difficult. Some of our authors work in settings as social workers, physicians, or chaplains where they have daily encounters with dementia. However, though most congregational clergy work with people or families with Alzheimer's disease, not every rabbi or cantor has personal dementia experiences in their own families. This book has required each contributor to dredge his or her own soul in order to find the channel for their expressions of this often painful subject. It is not an easy theme about which to write.

The book is divided into three sections, titled "Diagnosis," "Adaptation," and "Moving On," with several chapters in each division. Although the progression—or better, the regression—of Alzheimer's disease and dementia is not exactly linear, we have tried to capture a sense of flow with the themes of each chapter as they move successively in the ontology of the disease. Diagnosis often is a gray, loosely defined process, and similarly adaptation will vary from person to person and family to family. "Moving On" (a name brilliantly given to this section by Rabbi Richard Address as we sought to define the stages of the disease in a Jewish framework) seeks to offer the *nechemta* at the end of the process.

Opening the book is a sensitive foreword offered by Rabbi Simkha Y. Weintraub, who not only is the rabbinic director of the National

Jewish Healing Program in New York, working in every facet of Jewish healing, but also is pained by his own father's Alzheimer's disease. Thereafter, in the Diagnosis section, Beverly L. Engel and Cathy M. Lieblich, social workers respectively with the Alzheimer's Association and Pioneer Network, set the table, reminding the reader of the personhood of one with Alzheimer's disease and of the distinction between dementia and normal forgetfulness. Rabbi Jonathan V. Plaut then offers a profound and startling retrospective on his brilliant father, Rabbi W. Gunther Plaut, who struggled with his diagnosis of Alzheimer's disease. This is followed by a touching discussion of the role of family and community in giving support, written by Rabbi Paul J. Kipnes. Rabbi Bonnie Ann Steinberg, who serves as chaplain at a large nursing facility in the Bronx, New York, perceptively describes early responses to dementia in her chapter, which is followed by a review of Jewish halachic teachings bearing on the theme of Alzheimer's disease, prepared by Rabbi Elliot N. Dorff, rector of the American Jewish University in Los Angeles. The Diagnosis section concludes with rich chapters written by Cantor Ellen Dreskin, of Hebrew Union College–Jewish Institute of Religion in New York, about her own mother's experience with both blindness and dementia, and by Dr. Rhonna Shatz, chief of behavioral neurology at Henry Ford Hospital in Detroit, presenting both a history of Alzheimer's disease and a window into the brain itself, approached though texts from the Book of Genesis.

The second section, Adaptation, begins with "Doorways of Hope: Adapting to Alzheimer's," written by Rabbi Sheldon Marder of the Jewish Home in San Francisco, which offers a number of approaches for such adaptation. Thereafter, Mina Friedler, who conducts senior programming for the Jewish Center in Los Angeles, describes her own creative approaches, using art, music, dance, and intergenerational activities to engage persons with dementia. The section then continues with two soulful chapters, the first presenting a physician's per-

Editor's Note: Sadly, both Rabbi Jonathan V. Plaut and his father, Rabbi W. Gunther Plaut, each died as this book was nearing its completion, and the editor extends caring condolences to the Plaut family.

spective, sensitively written by Dr. Ronald M. Andiman, a neurologist in Los Angeles, and the second considering a new perspective on the disposition of the soul in persons with Alzheimer's disease, penned by Rabbi Michele B. Medwin. This section concludes with a treatise on memory and the Jew written by Rabbi Elyse Goldstein, stirred by thoughts of her own mother's living with Alzheimer's disease.

The book's final section, Moving On, is an encounter with the deeper losses experienced by those with Alzheimer's disease and dementia and by their caregivers. Its first chapter, by Dr. Toby F. Laping of SUNY Buffalo Medical School, reviews the processes, concerns, and timing of placing a family member in a care facility and ponders the teaching of the ancient sage Hillel, who taught, "If I am not for myself, who will be for me?" (*Pirkei Avot* 1:14). In "He's Still My Father," Rabbi Mike Comins describes a son's dilemmas in caring for his father, which is followed by a thoughtful look into the delicate area of spousal loyalty—if a spouse has dementia, is it adultery?—written by Rabbi Richard F. Address. I wrote the next chapter, questioning the nature of the soul and personhood in those who have Alzheimer's disease, and Rabbi Andrew Sklarz then describes the anguish of loss, written as he mourns his mother upon her death from the disease. Rabbi Cary Kozberg, a longtime chaplain at a large, Midwestern senior facility, concludes the volume with an important reminder of the abiding humanity of those with Alzheimer's disease, that even those who are broken fragments still retain their sacred humanness.

Supporting this book, from day one, has been the dedicated team at the URJ Press, led by its editor-in-chief, Michael Goldberg, to whom I extend my deepest appreciation. Michael's editorial insights improved the book immensely, and his calm, professional perspective and sure encouragement were sustaining comfort in the late hours when so much writing and editing took place. Moreover, his talented and conscientious staff—Jessica Katz, Fiorella deLima, Jonathan Levine, and Stephen Becker—helped in every step along the way and are the invisible but vital cogs in the Press's wonderful work. Much appreciation is due to the staff, leadership, and membership of my synagogue, Congregation Emanu El in Redlands, California, who took interest in and supported my efforts on this project. And, I extend my sincerest gratitude to colleagues, friends, and professionals in both the Jewish and the healing worlds to whom I turned for advice and suggestions, including Rabbis Richard Address, Eddie Feinstein, Dayle Friedman, Sid Helbraun, Alan Henkin, Jordan Parr, Hara Person, Debbie Prinz, Harry Rosenfeld, Ike Serotta, Simkha Weintraub, Eric Weiss, and Yoel Kahn, and Cantor Ellen Dreskin. Michele Prince, director of the Kalsman Institute for Judaism and Health, was instrumental in introducing me to key physicians. Similarly helpful were Sue Rosenthal of the National Center for Jewish Healing, and Karen Golden.

Finally, I offer insufficient appreciation to my family, who again surrendered me to the keyboard and the telephone at all hours of the day. My wife, Reva, thoughtfully listened to my thoughts and my frustrations and revisited the loss of her father as the volume unfolded. My children, Benjamin and Elena, though presently away at school, are hidden in the backstory of this book. With my father-in-law's diagnosis and developing illness, my wife and I determined in 1989 to change positions and relocate from western New York to nearer Philadelphia so we could assist in caregiving and provide our children some experience of their grandfather before it was too late. Thus, Alzheimer's disease reshaped the trajectory of my career and infused precious bonds in my family at the very time when loss was so imminent. I extend loving gratitude to Reva, Ben, and Elena for their support.

Yes, stone tablets and cherished lives can and do break. Often, only fragments remain. However, how we safeguard those enduring shards and derive unexpected meaning and value from the processes of living with such loss can very much define us and temper the disheartening experience. Years before there were MRIs or thirty-point questionnaires, the Talmudic Sages taught, "Respect the aged, because the fragments of the original tablets were preserved in the Ark with the new ones." Today, with our growing aged population, we need to be certain that the arks of our homes and our synagogues—and of our hearts and our minds—remain large and open to tenderly receive the living fragments of all our most cherished souls.

PART I

Diagnosis

1

꾝

Normal Forgetfulness, or . . .

Beverly L. Engel and Cathy M. Lieblich

To walk into a room and forget why you went there or occasionally to not be able to recall the name of someone you have known for years is an event universally experienced by people of all ages. As we grow older, these momentary lapses become more common and more disconcerting, often compelling us to laugh them off as "senior moments"—a popular term insinuating that advancing age is synonymous with mental decline. These brief moments of forgetfulness are quite anxiety provoking; yet, the physical signs of aging, such as graying hair, encroaching wrinkles, and deep-set lines, do not create the same sense of dread that our bodies are failing as do the occasional memory slips that make us think our minds may be betraying us.

The prospect of losing one's mind, and ultimately oneself, to Alzheimer's disease is what feeds the insecurities that are felt when a momentary lapse of memory occurs. Yet, even when unaffected by disease, there are normal changes in the brain that one might expect to experience. Knowing about these changes makes it easier to accept that, just like other parts of the body, the brain also naturally changes with age. The brain slows down, requiring more time to learn and store information. Recall or retrieval of information from the brain's mental storehouse also slows, reflecting the "it's on the tip of my tongue" phenomenon. Declines occur in working memory, the system the brain has for storing and manipulating information over a short period of time. (An example of working memory is holding a ten-digit telephone number in your head until you can write it down.) Distractions also are more likely to affect an older person's ability to concentrate, plus other changes can occur, including declines in reaction time.[1]

While many of these declines are understandably worrisome, they are not symptoms of Alzheimer's disease. However, identifying the signs of Alzheimer's disease is important, because recognizing these signs may lead to an early diagnosis, allowing valuable time for persons in the early stages of the disease to be involved in decisions that affect their own care and to be in control of their lives for as long as possible. A schematic developed by the Alzheimer's Association contrasts that which is normal forgetfulness due to aging with that which is abnormal or disease-based.[2]

SIGNS OF ALZHEIMER'S DISEASE	TYPICAL AGE-RELATED CHANGES
Poor judgment and [poor] decision making	Making a bad decision once in a while
Inability to manage a budget	Missing a monthly payment
Losing track of the date or season	Forgetting which day it is and remembering later
Difficulty having a conversation	Sometimes forgetting which word to use
Misplacing things and being unable to retrace steps to find them	Losing things from time to time

The most significant indication of Alzheimer's disease is when changes in memory and thinking impact or disrupt day-to-day activities, such as not being able to keep appointments, confusing days of the calendar, or not being able to complete tasks that once were second nature, like balancing a checkbook or starting a car. Imagine getting into a car with keys in hand, but still not understanding how to turn on the ignition. Such a challenge is indicative of the extent to which Alzheimer's impairs thinking.

The initial symptoms of Alzheimer's are mild, but because it is a progressive brain disorder that is fatal, decline is inevitable and ultimately causes an increased reliance on others for one's care. Experts have identified seven stages of the disease. This information, along with other hallmarks of the disease's progression, is widely publicized and is accessible at the website of the Alzheimer's Association, among other places. Elaborated below are the difficulties a person is likely to encounter early in the disease:

- Trouble planning and problem solving, staying organized, and following necessary steps to complete an activity, such as following a recipe.
- Misplacing items, such as putting the television remote in the microwave, and being unable to retrace one's steps in order to relocate items.
- Confusion over time and place, such as not knowing the season or the time of day, or not remembering how one arrived at a certain place, with disorientation likely even in familiar places.
- Social isolation and withdrawal from work or group activities. Social settings can be embarrassing and difficult to maneuver because of the inability to remember names or follow the flow of conversation or direction.
- Uncharacteristic mood or personality changes, such as paranoia, fearfulness, anger, aggression, withdrawal, or irritability. Personality changes arise as the individual tries to assert control in situations that are increasingly confusing. For example, a person who cannot find his wallet might accuse a family member of stealing it.
- Decreased or poor judgment, particularly when making financial decisions. The person with dementia may unwittingly give away large sums of money or become the victim of fraud or abuse.
- Trouble recognizing and understanding visual and spatial relationships. This often leads people to misinterpret what they see. A

throw rug may seem like a hole in the floor, or shadows may become scary.

- New problems with language and writing. Commonly, individuals cannot follow the train of conversation and may employ inaccurate or inappropriate word substitutions or non sequiturs. Handwriting becomes very small and illegible.

Despite these common manifestations of dementia, Alzheimer's disease is a highly individualized illness. It affects no two people in the same way. Not every person with the disease experiences all the symptoms associated with it. Despite this variability of symptoms, the disease has a relentless nature, and symptoms gradually worsen. Yet, it is important to recognize that the symptoms of the disease do not define, or redefine, the person. As care partners, our job, throughout the course of the disease, is to help our loved ones recognize their strengths and not focus on their disabilities. To do this effectively, care partners and persons with the diagnosis both must be willing to acknowledge and accept the changes that are occurring.

As caregivers to our own parents and as professionals in the field of aging, we, the coauthors, are keenly aware of the daily challenges families face as they struggle to provide the best care they can to their loved ones. For us, honoring our own, respective parents, including Beverly's father, who recently was diagnosed with Alzheimer's-type dementia, means helping them assert control over their lives for as long as possible. Through our own experiences, we realize that achieving this takes an intentional and conscious effort. When looking back at our own struggles, we know that our professional lives have informed our personal lives and helped us honor the people we knew, and know, our parents to be. This chapter illustrates how professional principles enlightened our paths as caregivers, and they may do the same for you.

When we face adverse events such as unwelcome news or unexpected change, the typical and immediate reaction often is not acceptance, as acknowledgment of new, difficult realities is exhaustingly emotional work. Recently in one of our offices, a woman in her late seventies explained that her family insisted she was forgetful, and she needed to see a physician regarding her memory. The woman was convinced that nothing was wrong, and she refused to acknowledge her family's concerns. It wasn't until later in the week, when her car needed gasoline, that she suddenly realized her family's assertions were correct. Standing in front of the gasoline pump, knowing her car was on empty, she found her mind a complete blank. Unable to figure out how to use the apparatus, she stood staring at the pump and then at the car. Finally, with panic rising in her stomach, she got back in her car and drove home without filling her gas tank. This incident is what changed her denial into disbelief, shock, and grief. It was the defining moment that allowed her to move on. Though still not fully accepting of what was happening to her, it enabled her to take the next step to arrange for a thorough medical evaluation.

Biblical and historical references to transitions in Jewish life document the difficulty of accepting change. Psalm 137:1, "By the rivers of Babylon, there we sat, sat and wept, as we thought of Zion," depicts the shock and grief felt by the Jewish people upon their dispersion into exile after the destruction of the First Temple by the Babylonians. Torn from their homes, their families, and the life they had once known, these Jews were forced to face a questionable future. Weeping, mourning, and promising not to forget their precious city, Jerusalem, they began their eventual transition from disbelief and immobility to accepting a new, though not preferred, station in life. For persons with Alzheimer's disease and their families, the journey toward acceptance is similar.

Ignoring the signs of memory loss is a way families initially cope with what seems unimaginable: the loss of a loved one to a disease that eradicates memory and cognitive function. To deny a problem exists not only excuses family members from having to assume caregiver responsibility, but enables them to live in the present without worrying about the unpredictability of the future. What appears to be the shirking of caregiving responsibility is actually a coping mechanism that allows time for an adjustment to a new reality.

On the other side, the looming fear within people facing Alzheimer's disease is the prospect of losing themselves to the ravages of the disease. This woeful and overwhelming fear of not remembering who one is or that which was important in life is embodied by Psalm 137:5, "If I forget you, O Jerusalem, let my right hand wither." By lamenting their displacement from Jerusalem, the exiled Jews were aware that they might forget their homeland and lose the strong connection that they had had to the land; their physical proximity on the land is what defined their peoplehood. Like Jews in that time of exile, persons in the very early stages of Alzheimer's are similarly terrified at the prospect that they will no longer remember who they are and what is significant to them. Their future, which once was bright, now looks dismal, with expectations for loss dotting the horizon.

Of course, some people with the disease may actually forget that they forget, but for those who do recognize their symptoms, denial is a strong and complicated coping mechanism. Denial can materialize before or after a diagnosis, it can be either a temporary or long-term condition, and it can occur for all sorts of reasons. People in the early stages of the disease may deny their symptoms because their lapses of memory are too distressing. Sometimes people in denial think that if they ignore what is unpleasant, it eventually will go away. Others fear the stigma associated with having Alzheimer's disease and worry that family and friends will ostracize them. Whatever the reason, denial is not to be construed as intentional behavior meant to frustrate care partners, but as a natural response to behavioral symptoms that are abnormal and unsettling.

In order to best plan for the future, moving past the denial phase is vastly important. Care partners typically grasp the reality of Alzheimer's before the person who has the disease does so; thus, the question is this: How might family members help the person accept the diagnosis and learn to live with its ongoing challenges? To get past denial, families can take part in an ongoing conversation that engages all players and initially assures the person with dementia that he or she is cared for and will continue to be cared for. Over time, communication, love, patience, and understanding are the best approaches to convincing the diagnosed person to seek medical advice, to cultivate support from others, and to find new ways to cope with changing symptoms.

Organizing a supportive team that works well together brings a sense of relief to the person in the early stages of dementia, as well as to family caregivers. The more support there is, the less likely a person with dementia will have to persevere alone and the less likely a care partner will have to singularly shoulder the full responsibility of care. While a care team may be composed of a range of persons, including a spouse, adult children, extended family members, close friends, physicians, counselors, and other supportive community service professionals, what makes a care team successful is when the person in the early stage of Alzheimer's disease is assisted to participate in and make decisions about his or her own care for as long as possible.

We have learned that it is critically important to have a care team in place that can assist the person with Alzheimer's disease to plan for the future while he or she can still express preferences and wishes for future care options. Yet, because of the tendency to err on the side of safety, one pitfall into which caregivers often fall is to make unilateral decisions on behalf of the person who is in the early stages of the disease without consulting or conferring with him or her. These unilateral decisions almost always concern some manner of restricting activity, and for the person in the early stages of dementia, these decisions can appear hurtful and controlling. For example, a person in these early stages may insist that he or she can still drive effectively, while family members are pushing to take the car away. Such decisions that restrict activity should not be made subjectively, which is why broaching such subjects, like driving, with one's neurologist or another specialist can bring new information to a discussion. Being able to obtain objective opinions from doctors and community support personnel helps the care team make informed decisions that are less emotionally subjective. In this instance, a physician might suggest actual parameters the family can use to judge the driving ability of a person with dementia. Thereafter, the person who refuses to stop driving might agree to stop if the family documents unsafe activities as described by the physician. For instance, these parameters may include whether the driver stays in the proper lane, stops and starts in moving traffic, drives significantly more slowly than the speed limit, or loses the way while driving. In this way, by consulting the physician or other professional, the person with memory loss can be assured that his or her independence is not being restricted arbitrarily.

It is so important not to exclude or marginalize the person with dementia, especially as the disease progresses. Too often, persons with dementia find themselves, either by choice or by circumstance, left out of conversations, social situations, and even decisions about their own lives. This pushes them further into withdrawal, silence, and depression. And, even the reverse is seen, where challenging and difficult behaviors become the expressed form of fighting back to retain the independence and connectedness they see slipping away.

This sense of loss is comparable to the experience of the Jews who were expelled from the Kingdom of Judah in 586 BCE. Those in the early stage of Alzheimer's disease, who are witnessing the familiar become unfamiliar, as well as their caregivers, may feel like they too have entered into a strange, new territory. The Jews who were forced into foreign lands and required to worship foreign gods thought that they would lose their connection to their own God. They lamented in Psalm 137:4, "How can we sing a song of the LORD on alien soil?" Yet, compelled to live in a strange land without knowing their future, they could not imagine how transformative their anguish, hopelessness, and despair eventually would be for the Jewish people as a whole. What actually happened was that these Jews were indeed able to sing a new song in a foreign land by discovering that they could still be faithful to their own monotheistic beliefs in a strange place. Out of despair came new insights about how life could be restructured and begun anew in a new place without displacing core religious beliefs. In effect, their anguish led to the development of the Diaspora, where vibrant centers of Jewish life flourished for centuries outside of the ancient Kingdom of Judah.[3]

How does this translate to persons with dementia and their caregivers? How do caregivers sing a new song in a foreign land? One way is to remember that persons with dementia deserve every opportunity for a life that has meaning, regardless of their level of memory impairment. If, as caregivers, we are charged with upholding our loved one's abiding personhood, then it is incumbent upon us to preserve the value and worth of that person through love, patience, understanding, compassion, acceptance, and affirmation of his or her identity.

Tom Kitwood, an innovator in the field of dementia care and the author of *Dementia Reconsidered: The Person Comes First,* writes about the four "global states" of well-being: *personal worth,* or a feeling of self-esteem and personal value; *agency,* or a sense of having some control over one's personal life; *social confidence,* or a feeling of being at ease in the company of others; and *hope,* which is a general sense that the future will be good.[4] These principles can transform the relationship between care partners and the person with Alzheimer's disease. Although receiving a diagnosis of Alzheimer's disease is hard and being a caregiver to someone with progressive memory loss is infinitely challenging, undertaking these challenges in a way that boosts family relationships, eases tensions, uplifts the spirit, and affirms the human condition can offer opportunities for meaningful and satisfying times together and may diminish the chaos and terror that can be the downward spiral of Alzheimer's disease.

One might ask how these global traits described by Kitwood are expressed in day-to-day interactions between the caregiver and the care recipient. To ensure personal worth, it is important to focus on the person's abilities as opposed to the disabilities. We urge caregivers to allow and encourage their family member with dementia to do everything he or she can do for as long as possible. Even if eating finger foods with one's hands is messy and takes a long time, it is more of an independent act than being fed by someone else. Another way to ensure personal worth is to honor the family member and keep the essence of his or her individualism intact. Caregivers become memory keepers, preserving their loved one's life story. When acting on behalf of a loved one with Alzheimer's, caregivers should endeavor to recognize and respect their loved one's desires, preferences, and likes and dislikes.

To maintain agency, or the sense of having control over one's personal life, people with Alzheimer's disease should continue to have a voice for as long as possible in how they want their care delivered. As a caregiver, never assume that the type of care you want is the same as that which your family member may want. Talk about future plans together. Prepare now for the day when long-term care services may be needed. These conversations are best conducted when the person with dementia is in the early stages of the disease and can still express preferences for care. A board-certified elder law attorney can help families facilitate these conversations and assist with legal and financial planning.

Another way to exert control over one's life is to indulge in activities that are meaningful and pleasurable. Beverly's dad still plays bridge. Occasionally he forgets the rules of the game, but he is lucky enough to play with a group of men who gently remind him how to play. Sometimes, his weekly games put a little bit of money in his pocket, but more importantly, he enjoys the social interaction with friends and the time spent with a lifelong hobby. Involvement in enjoyable and validating activities is more significant than the type of activity, especially when those activities enhance an individual's self-esteem and the time spent doing them is perceived as worthwhile. The process of involvement in an activity is far more important than the outcome or product of the activity.

Interestingly, this idea of enabling the person with Alzheimer's disease to maintain agency and a measure of control over his or her personal life may appear contrary to Psalm 137. In the psalm, we read, "If I forget you, O Jerusalem, let my right hand wither" (137:5). Clearly, the biblical penalty of forgetting was to suffer personal loss of ability, whereas memory was the mechanism for retaining competency and personal agency. However, today we would suggest that when memory goes, and so ebbs one's self-reliance, it is exactly the time to do all that we can, as care partners, in order to retain the self-will of our family member. From our ancient exiles and the text of the psalm, we have learned the awful sadness of surrender and loss; therefore we should do whatever we can to obviate it in our day.

For most people, social confidence comes with being in the company of others. Yet, those with Alzheimer's may feel sidelined by their friends, or they may withdraw from social gatherings because they are too self-conscious about exposing their cognitive losses in a social setting. Yet staying connected to old friends or finding new friends who understand the circumstances of Alzheimer's disease improves social well-being. How do individuals with Alzheimer's and their caregivers maintain social connections? One possibility is to explain the situation to close friends. Tell them how valued their continued friendship is at this time, and give them specific ways that contact can be maintained. One example might be to replace telephone conversations that are becoming too difficult with a weekly lunch date, in which face-to-face conversations are easier. Sometimes nothing that one may do or say will make a difference, and old friends may drop out of sight. In this instance, it is best to replace old friends with new friends. Find an early-stage support group where you and your loved one can meet others in the same situation as yourselves. Often, it is on the basis of shared experiences that friendships are formed.

Irrespective of how one maintains social contact, there are several important points to remember. The more a person with Alzheimer's disease is socially engaged, the more he or she will practice language skills and perhaps delay the "if you don't use it, you'll lose it" condition. Secondly, large group gatherings can be overwhelming when multiple conversations occur at once. It is preferable to engage in small social gatherings where the conversation is intimate and the ability to handle incoming stimuli is not compromised. We all enjoy being with people who make us feel good about ourselves and in whose company we are comfortable, and this is particularly true for people with Alzheimer's disease.

Even if the person with memory loss cannot recall recent experiences or if what happens today is not remembered tomorrow, the goal for the person with Alzheimer's disease is to still enjoy the moment, to live in the present, to laugh with family and friends, and to enjoy companionship. This is the higher purpose of being socially engaged, and in the end, it is these moments that give the person with memory loss, and caregivers, hope for the future and offer assurances that there are still good days ahead.

When we start down the caregiving journey, we surely can't predict what the experience will be like. As caregivers, we never know what transformative experiences and blessings may come from being thrust into an unfamiliar caregiving role, like the unexpected outcomes of the exiled Israelites in the sixth century BCE. While Beverly was growing up, her father occasionally said he loved her. Now that he is diagnosed with Alzheimer's, he tells her every time they speak that he loves her. Toward the end of Cathy's mother's life, she often needed to rest in bed, which gave Cathy the opportunity to lie in bed with her and share a physical closeness that they might not otherwise have had. For us, these increased levels of intimacy were unexpected gifts. Other caregivers may find gifts in other places. They might recognize positive attributes in themselves, such as patience and understanding. They might take on roles that they never expected, such as grandchildren who willingly and lovingly assist with a grandparent's care. These unanticipated and challenging experiences in life mold us into our best selves.

There is something meaningful about being transformed by the experience. If caregivers strive to uphold Kitwood's four global traits, which we refer to as the four commandments of caregiving—personal worth, agency, social confidence, and hope—then transforming experiences that change our understanding of ourselves, of the person we care for, and of the bond between caregiver and care receiver are bound to occur.

2

❧

Recognizing Changes

JONATHAN V. PLAUT

"Rabbi, today we are going to see the doctor," said Ray, my father's most caring and attentive caregiver. "Eat your breakfast, Rabbi, and then we will get ready to go to the doctor," Ray reminded him with a gentle touch.

"Today is Wednesday?" Dad queried.

"Yes, Rabbi, today is Wednesday, and we have a ten o'clock appointment with the doctor," Ray responded.

"Wednesday, November 10," Dad muttered under his breath as he glanced at the *Globe and Mail* lying on the table before him. As he ate his cereal, he continued in near silence for a few moments and then looked again at Ray for confirmation, "Jean Chrétien is the prime minister, and we live in Toronto." He stared at Ray, hoping he was correct.

"Yes, Rabbi," Ray responded rather anxiously as he waited for him to finish his breakfast. Dad nodded and under his breath he recited, "Glass, table, lamp"—three words the doctor always asked him to remember. He recited almost inaudibly a sentence using the three

Editor's Note: Sadly, both Rabbi Jonathan V. Plaut and his father, Rabbi W. Gunther Plaut, each died as this book was nearing its completion, and the editor extends caring condolences to the Plaut family.

words as the doctor always asked him to do at the appointment. "The glass was sitting on the table by the lamp."

"Okay, Rabbi, we need to get dressed now and drive to our appointment," Ray said as he guided my father to his bedroom. But Dad was notably lost in thought as Ray helped dress him.

After a short time in the waiting room, my sister, Judith, and I, along with my father and his caregivers, Ray and Arlene, entered the doctor's office.

"Hello, Rabbi," the doctor called out in a very warm welcome to him.

"Shalom," the rabbi responded quite nonchalantly. The four of us took chairs behind my father but said nothing to the doctor. After a few moments, the doctor began his thirty-point, quarterly assessment.

"Rabbi," the doctor asked him, "what is today?"

"Wednesday," he responded.

"The date, Rabbi?" the doctor inquired.

"November 10," the rabbi answered. The doctor continued to run through his questions and gave him the three words, "glass, table, and lamp," to remember in a few minutes. The doctor continued his questions, which included asking for the name of the prime minister of Canada.

"Jean Chrétien," Dad responded quickly.

"Where do you live, Rabbi?" the doctor rambled on with his list of questions.

"Toronto."

"Now Rabbi, give me the three words I told you about a short time ago." Dad rattled off the three words without a moment's hesitation.

"Glass, table, and lamp," he said.

"Can you make a sentence?" the doctor asked.

Dad sat in deep thought. "On the table by the lamp is a glass," he responded quite proudly.

"Good, Rabbi," said the doctor as he completed the test. Dad smiled broadly, knowing he had done a good job. The doctor looked at the four of us and said, "I am amazed, as again the rabbi had twenty-eight correct out of thirty, and that is unheard of with his disease." My father was always competitive and most accustomed to taking tests. When the doctor finally listened to our pleas to deviate from the usual test format and ask a few different questions, my father's test score dropped to eighteen out of thirty.

Many would call Rabbi W. Gunther Plaut one of the greatest Reform Jewish scholars of the twentieth century. He was a prolific writer; he authored twenty-five books, published more than a thousand articles, wrote a weekly column for thirty years in the *Canadian Jewish News*, and was a regular contributor to the Toronto *Globe and Mail* in addition to other newspapers and magazines, two encyclopedias, and many anthologies and learned journals. His writings include works on theology, philosophy, and even two books of historical fiction. His most acclaimed publications, used by Reform congregations around the world, are *The Torah: A Modern Commentary* and *The Haftarah Commentary*. My father was a renaissance man who was a leading authority on Reform Judaism and a passionate supporter of numerous human rights causes. He traveled extensively throughout the world as a frequent scholar-in-residence.

W. Gunther Plaut was born in 1912 in the small university town of Munster, Westphalia, in the western part of Germany, a short distance from the Dutch border. His father, Jonas Plaut, was a teacher at a local Jewish seminary; his mother was a native of Munster. The family remained there until the coming of the Nazi regime forced them to emigrate. My father grew up in a rather solitary manner within the confines of the orphanage that his parents administered. In 1930, he became the youngest student to enter the University of Berlin Law School, and three years later, he obtained a doctorate in jurisprudence. With the Nazis having seized power, my father realized he would never be able to pursue a legal career in Germany. His father suggested he study Hebrew with Rabbi Abraham Joshua Heschel at the Berlin Institute for Jewish Studies, where he also took courses taught by Dr. Leo Baeck, who at the time was the chief rabbi of the city of Berlin.

In the spring of 1935, Dr. Baeck received a letter from the president of the Hebrew Union College in Cincinnati, Dr. Julian Morgenstern, which offered to enroll five "capable and promising young German students who are now preparing for the Rabbinate in Germany but who may desire for one reason or another, to continue their studies at the Hebrew Union College." At the urging of his parents, Gunther Plaut accepted Dr. Morgenstern's invitation and left for the United States of America to begin his new life.

In Cincinnati, he met Elizabeth Strauss, whom he married on November 10, 1938. He was unaware of the fact that while he was getting married, all the synagogues of Germany were being torched and that his father had gone into hiding. The date of my parents' wedding became known as *Kristallnacht*—the Night of Broken Glass.

Ordained in 1939 at the Hebrew Union College, my father's first pulpit was in Chicago as an assistant rabbi. The position afforded him the opportunity to spend some time in scholarly pursuits. He became contributing editor in Bible for the *Universal Jewish Encyclopaedia* and also wrote for various journals. In 1943, a few days after becoming an American citizen, my father enlisted in the Chaplain Corps of the United States Army. He was shipped overseas as a chaplain with the 104th Infantry Division, where he saw combat and witnessed the opening of the first concentration camp. The recipient of the Bronze Star for his war service, my father left the army in 1946, returned to Chicago, and continued his scholarly pursuits.

In 1948 my father became rabbi of Mount Zion Temple in Saint Paul, Minnesota, where he served for thirteen years. During that period, he published his first books on history and Bible. He became involved in the political life of the community, becoming a close friend to many who would later make their mark in national politics, including Herbert Humphrey, Walter Mondale, Eugene McCarthy, and Orville Freeman.

In 1961, he went to Toronto to become the senior rabbi at Holy Blossom Temple. There he became the undisputed leader of the Jewish community and, in time, the voice of Canadian Jewry. In 1977, just before he chose to retire, he became president of the Canadian Jewish Congress and in 1981 the president of the Central Conference of American Rabbis.

My father's main reason for leaving the active rabbinate was his desire to finish his magnum opus, *The Torah: A Modern Commentary*.

Published in 1981, the commentary quickly attained international acclaim. In 1996, he published a commentary on the haftarah. His Torah and haftarah commentaries, published in one volume by the Reform Movement in 2005, are a lasting tribute to his superb scholarship and are his lasting legacy.

And then, Rabbi W. Gunther Plaut, with arguably one of the greatest minds in the Reform rabbinate, would be diagnosed with Alzheimer's disease.

How did my father deal with the new changes that Alzheimer's disease would inflict on his everyday life? He was extremely fortunate to have two wonderful caregivers, Ray and Arlene Oliveros, who helped him adjust to his new norm.

My father's active life as a rabbi meant that he became accustomed to always having a schedule in order to cope with the demands on his time. Each day, in keeping with this habit, he would ask Ray and Arlene, "What's on the agenda?" and Ray and Arlene would have to tell him, repeatedly, the plans for that day. They might include going to Holy Blossom Temple to pick up his mail or out for a drive. The caregivers realized early on that variety in his daily activities was a major part of maintaining his well-being.

Each morning, my father still worked at his computer to write an article, prepare a speech, or work on his latest manuscript. Secretly, however, Ray would go on the computer beforehand and introduce grammatical and spelling errors. He would then suggest to my father that he look at the article he wrote and make sure that everything was written properly. My father would then sit at the computer for several hours reading the manuscript and making corrections to the document that Ray had already corrupted. Upon finishing the task, my father would comment that he felt productive because he had worked on his new manuscript. This activity continued for many months until it became apparent that my father could no longer make corrections and that he had lost his ability to use the computer.

My father still attended Shabbat services regularly and sat in the pews singing parts of the songs and melodies he knew so well, looking at the words that ever so slowly seemed to become unrecognizable to him. He felt comfortable when congregants would come up to him to say hello and to receive from him a smile or wave, which made them presume, erroneously, that he knew who they were. His weekly attendance at services gave him some of his old identification as a rabbi.

In the early stages of his illness, Ray and Arlene were most gracious and invited guests to the home for dinner on Friday nights. While it was already difficult for my father to carry on a meaningful conversation, there were moments of enlightenment when he would utter a knowledgeable comment that would silence the others at the table. Unfortunately, as time progressed, he sat with a distant, vacant stare as the blessings were recited by my sister and me.

As a lifelong avid athlete, my father required daily exercise for his mental and physical health. He had been an outstanding tennis player from his youth, and he regularly enjoyed the game throughout his life, even superseding his pleasure in playing golf. The physical demands of playing tennis worked to keep his endorphins at a reasonable level, so Ray and Arlene would drive him several times a week to the tennis club, where he would play with the pro. Many other players at the club would watch him through the visitors' window, marveling at how he was still able to volley with the pro. He was always delighted when tennis was included in his daily schedule. This activity continued for quite some time, until his inability to walk ended his tennis career.

During the summer months, Ray took my father to play golf. Ray would encourage my father to play a few holes, and when he tired after two or three holes, they would meet Arlene and occasionally my sister, Judith, and have lunch. He seemed to be more alert and would enjoy a better lunch when he was out in public. He enjoyed that many club members would stop by his table to greet him.

My father also had been a chess player all of his life. He had even published a few chess problems in addition to his other academic writings. My father and Ray would sit and play chess in those early days after diagnosis, when my father's competitive nature made him always interested in winning.

Finally, my father attended a social justice program sponsored by Holy Blossom Temple each Thursday evening, from November through the middle of April. The program was called "Out of the Cold," and it helped feed and house the homeless, one evening a week, during the winter months. Ray and Arlene took him to meet and greet the "guests," sit with them, eat dinner, and interact to the best of his abilities. The guests were always happy to see him, and he continued to attend the program for several years. By attending, he also received a warm welcome from his old congregants working the program.

Ray and Arlene helped to provide my father with a good quality of life in spite of his limitations. Dad wanted to be active, and they kept him involved throughout the day. As time unfolded, these activities also came to an end; but for some years, he was able to be out and about, living life to the fullest—based on his ability.

My father showed how strong-willed and determined he was as he attempted to overcome Alzheimer's. Using his superb intellect, he tried to fool others, yet he did not realize others knew his mental capabilities were not the same as before. Many people he met swore that he knew who they were, even though we knew he had no idea. When someone had the audacity to ask him to tell her her name, he would quip immediately, "Well, my dear lady, of course I know you." He had an amazing ability to cover his impairment, which he did for many months.

Throughout my father's life, he had a routine, which included writing early in the morning. By midmorning, he concluded his writing and continued with his daily activities. He certainly realized that his writing had deteriorated, as my father was always honest about himself and his human frailties. In his final article in the *Canadian Jewish News*, he concluded writing more than thirty years of weekly articles for the paper, voicing his philosophy, and ultimately, revealing his illness in a most moving fashion. This farewell to the thousands of people who read his weekly musings crystallized in many ways his philosophy of life.

He wrote:

> One of the fundamental experiences of being human is being subject to physical and mental problems. Rabbis are no exception.
>
> I don't hesitate to tell you that last month I celebrated my ninety-first birthday, which means I still have a long way to go

if I am to equal my mother's journey. From her I learned that getting old does not necessarily mean wilting away like a dying flower, but now that I am old, I realize that I once took for granted that the youthful alertness of my own mind would last forever and hopefully be paralleled by my physical capacity.

I had passed my ninetieth birthday and at first everything seemed to remain the same. But then, one problem after another began to assail me. But that was minor, of course, compared to what happened to my beloved Elizabeth, my mate of sixty-five wonderful and productive years. As you know, she became ill several years ago and was finally claimed by the Angel of Death only a few months ago. Her illness and now her death have left me in a state of desolation that I have never before experienced.

In addition, I have come to feel in this last while that I was strangely debilitated. Not only did I have physical problems—I had expected them—but my mind too was not functioning with its usual alacrity. I did not seem to be able to make decisions, and when I finally made them, I often did not carry them out. I did not know why this was happening, and therefore sought medical help.

The diagnosis was that I now suffer, like many people my age—and some younger—from Alzheimer's disease. And I want you, my friends and readers, to know this straight from me, I will continue to do my best, but my best is no longer what it once was. So, like everyone else, regardless of age or health, I now face a basic question: how exactly can I do my best in waging a battle against Alzheimer's disease and, of course, for life?

The answer, simple though it may seem, is best expressed by the brief Hebrew expression *chazak v'ematz*. I will attempt to be as strong as possible and muster up as much courage as possible, knowing that much has been given to me in life, and knowing, as well, that much is in the hands of the Almighty.

And, my friends, I would say the same to you in whatever battle you must wage for life and for health: *chazak v'ematz*, be strong and be of good courage, and may you and I be granted the privilege of living for as long as our strength and God afford us.[1]

My father faced the onset of his disease directly by doing his best. In Canada, yearly driving tests are mandatory for those over eighty years of age. Passing the test each year seemed a given for my father until his ninety-first birthday, when he failed the test. He was told he could pay a substantial fee for a reassessment from a firm that handled appeals. Not wanting to lose his independence, he insisted that he would appeal this decision. But when he was reexamined, the results confirmed the decision. Visibly upset when he returned home, I said to him, "What are you so upset about? Now you have Ray's wife, Arlene, to drive you wherever you want. And, you do not have to worry about getting wet when it rains."

His face suddenly exhibited a broad smile. "I have a driver now," he uttered and showed me two thumbs-up. While he seemed to accept the fact that he could no longer drive, he continued to stubbornly insist for some months that he carry the car keys in his pocket.

As a competitive person all his life, he recognized the changes to his mental alacrity; but he fought to continue his regular routine even though the changes were abundantly obvious even to him, though he hoped maybe not to others. So he attempted to fool the doctor, and because the doctor did not vary his thirty-point quiz, the doctor was indeed baffled by my father's abilities in spite of the disease. He studied for the doctor's test each quarter, just as he did for all the challenges he experienced in life—whether preparing for a lecture, a sermon, a eulogy for a congregant, or a major address before ten thousand people.

My father faced the disease directly, by telling others honestly about it. When it was clear that his weekly article in the *Canadian Jewish News* was ending, he told his readers about his disease. The great Mishnaic sage Hillel used to say, B'makom she-ein anashim, hishtadeil lih'yot ish, "In a place where there is no humanity, strive to be human" (*Pirkei Avot* 2:5). My father tried desperately to retain his humanity even as his mind, and later his body, seemed to betray him. But humanity for my father included being honest and forthright about his age and stage in life. Humanity was not just about living as a human with one's mental and physical abilities; "striving to be human" meant facing the future in the same manner.

My father exemplified the dictum "Be strong and of good courage"— *Chazak v'ematz* (I Chronicles 28:20). He faced death with strength and courage. In the last television interview my father gave, in 2002 on a CBC program with Evan Solomon, he was asked about death and dying. I recall my father's short summary of his life: "I have lived a charmed life. I have survived the Nazis. I have survived the war; and I have been in extraordinary health. I have never been ill in my life; and I have full command of my mental and reasonable command of my physical capacities. Sooner or later, I have to expect to die anyway. Maybe a little sooner or later—who knows?" For him, "the fear of death was zero," and at nearly ninety years of age when the interview occurred, he knew "that death was down the road." But, when it would occur or how it would unfold, he left to the hands of the One above. He felt the Almighty had blessed him, and whatever the future held for him, he was prepared for it.

There is a great Chasidic tale that may help us understand how my father felt about life:

Some Chasidim of the Maggid of Mezheritz came to him. "Rebbe, we are puzzled. It says in the Talmud that we must thank God as much for the bad days as for the good. How can that be? What would our gratitude mean if we gave it equally for the good and the bad?"

The Maggid replied, "Go to Anapol. Reb Zusya will have an answer for you."

The Chasidim undertook the journey. Arriving in Anapol, they inquired for Reb Zusya. At last, they came to the poorest street of the city. There, crowded between two small houses, they found a tiny shack, sagging with age.

When they entered, they saw Reb Zusya sitting at a bare table, reading a volume by the light of the only small window. "Welcome, strangers!" he said. "Please pardon me for not getting up; I have hurt my leg. Would you like food? I have some bread. And there is water!"

"No. We have come only to ask you a question. The Maggid of Mezheritz told us you might help us understand: why do our Sages tell us to thank God as much for the bad days as for the good?"

Reb Zusya laughed. "Me? I have no idea why the Maggid sent you to me." He shook his head in puzzlement. "You see, I have never had a bad day. Every day God has given to me has been filled with miracles."

My father escaped the Nazis and had to make a new life in a strange land, so, for him, as for Reb Zusya, every day was a blessing. Finally, my father believed firmly that the future challenges he would face with his newly diagnosed Alzheimer's disease must rest in the hands of the Almighty. Once again, there is a famous Chasidic tale about Zusya that fits my father's philosophy of life:

Once, the great Chasidic leader Zusya came to his followers. His eyes were red with tears, and his face was pale with fear. "Zusya, what's the matter? You look frightened!" the befuddled disciples asked the wise sage.

"The other day, I had a vision. In it, I learned the question that the angels will one day ask me about my life," he replied.

The followers were puzzled. "Zusya, you are pious. You are scholarly and humble. You have helped so many of us. What question about your life could be so terrifying that you would be frightened to answer it?"

Zusya turned his gaze to heaven. "I have learned that the angels will not ask me, 'Why weren't you a Moses, leading your people out of slavery?'"

His followers persisted. "So, what will they ask you?"

"And I have learned," Zusya sighed, "that the angels will not ask me, 'Why weren't you a Joshua, leading your people into the Promised Land?'"

One of his followers approached Zusya and placed his hands on Zusya's shoulders. Looking him in the eyes, the follower demanded, "But what will they ask you?"

"They will say to me, 'Zusya, there was only one thing that no power of heaven or earth could have prevented you from becoming.' They will say, 'Zusya, why weren't you Zusya?'"

What do we learn from facing changes in life? We come to understand that as life changes constantly, one has to be honest about them. When one is unable to produce at the same level as one did before, it is important to admit this reality not just to oneself, but to others. We learn that courage to accept the changes can be difficult, but we have no choice but to do so. *Da lifnei mi atah omeid*, "Know before whom you stand." We all stand before the Almighty. Ultimately, everything is in God's hands. My father knew before whom he stood and was strong as he entered this final stage in his life. Like the lesson in our Chasidic tale, my father tried to be true to himself.

Now I, too, face challenges that will bring me to the end of my life, maybe even before my father's. There is much I can learn from my father and our Jewish texts as I battle my own illness and fate, amyotrophic lateral sclerosis (ALS, or Lou Gehrig's disease). I hope to have the courage and strength, with the help of the Almighty, to live as fully as possible, even as my muscles continue to weaken. How ironic that my father's keen mind has been taken from him while his muscles remain, whereas my mind will remain intact as my muscles are permanently lost. There is an old German expression: *Der Mensch denkt und Gott lenkt*, "Man proposes and God disposes." The future is not in our hands, only the manner in which we accept or embrace our finitude.

As my father said, "*Chazak v'ematz*—be strong and be of good courage!"

3

⚜

Remembering Grandma Esther: Community as Support and Validation

PAUL J. KIPNES

I have vivid memories of visiting my grandmother Esther at the home that she and my Grandpa Eddie shared in Framingham, Massachusetts. I knew enough to eat a light breakfast on those mornings. Esther came from that denomination of Judaism that equated providing food with showing love. One afternoon, Grandma suggested a tuna fish sandwich and some blueberries and sour cream for lunch. While she prepared food in the kitchen, I sat in the dining room, and we called out to each other. Grandma Esther always seemed to enjoy asking questions, and she delighted in hearing about anything and everything. We talked about school, my life, and with whom I was staying for the weekend. I am not sure she was able to keep straight which of my friends was whom, but I quickly learned that it did not really matter to her. It was the company—the time together—that was meaningful.

Moments later, she brought out a bagel with a shmear of cream cheese and some sliced bananas. Thinking that she had forgotten the meal we had agreed upon, I said, "Grandma, I was going to have a tuna fish sandwich and some blueberries and sour cream. Did you forget?" With the most loving look on her smiling face, she reassured me that she didn't forget. "No, this is just to tide you over while I make your lunch." In the span of a short hour and a half, I ate two meals that day, just to make Grandma happy. So began a ritual that would fatten me up over the next few years.

That Friday afternoon I learned a few significant lessons that would carry me through my rabbinical career: that the things we talk about are often less important than the time we spend together; that sometimes the most significant gift we can give to another person is our precious presence; and that when visiting with another person, be prepared to eat way more than one planned. And, that Alzheimer's disease—which took Esther's life away—ravages both the patient herself and her immediate family and the communities to which she belongs.

Creating Community

Esther Kipnes, my grandmother, lived much of her adult life in Framingham and Dorchester, small towns near Boston, Massachusetts. There, with her husband, my grandpa Eddie, she created a home and filled it with delicious smells and warm welcomes. Every holiday, she brought together her community—usually consisting of her two adult children, their spouses and families, her elderly parents, Bubbe and Papa, and a smattering of other relatives—to bless, eat, and celebrate. It was this community, eventually decreased by the parents and husband predeceasing her, but increased by the many spouses and grandchildren who entered their lives, that would suffer greatly as Esther began to suffer the effects of Alzheimer's disease. It was also this community that would have benefited from a community approach to caring for people with Alzheimer's disease.

In *Pirkei Avot* (the Teachings of Our Ancestors), our Talmudic Rabbis urge us, *Al tifrosh min hatzibur*, "Do not separate yourself from the community" (4:5). So important to Jewish life is communal connection that almost every life-cycle event requires the presence of a minyan of ten Jewish adults. A minyan gathers to witness a wedding, to hear the bar or bat mitzvah chant Torah, and, some say, to welcome a child into the covenant with God (though there is debate as to whether a minyan is necessary for the *b'rit milah* since proof of this event is marked upon the baby boy's body). Following the death of a loved one, the community brings itself to the mourners' home— for shivah, seven days and nights of intense mourning—to ensure that the mourners have a minyan to say *Kaddish* and have food to sustain themselves at the very moment when they have no desire to eat. A minyan then gathers together a year later to mark the *yahrzeit*, the anniversary of death. In celebration of life and in mourning a death, Jews are commanded to gather in community. Again, the Talmudic Rabbis, in *Mishnah Pei-ah* 1:1, remind us that every Jew is expected to assemble to celebrate, study, or mourn when members of the community need them.

But what are we supposed to do with and for people with Alzheimer's disease, whose lives, and the lives of those who love them, balance somewhere between life and death in an increasingly degenerative cycle? What are the family and communal obligations regarding a loved one who is physically alive, but whose mind and memory are slowly dying?

Remembering and Forgetting

Jews are keenly aware of the power of remembering. Shabbat, our weekly holy day, is welcomed with two candles: one each to remember the two different articulations in the Torah of the commandment of Shabbat. One candle is lit for *shamor*, the commandment in Exodus to "keep" Shabbat, while the other is for *zachor*, the command in Deuteronomy to "remember" Shabbat. We sing *L'chah Dodi*, saying *Shamor v'zachor b'dibur echad* ("Keep" and "remember": a single command), recalling the tradition that these two words were recited simultaneously in one divine utterance. It teaches that by remembering we keep Shabbat observance alive, and through Shabbat observance, we keep our people alive.

On the most sacred of our holy days, Yom Kippur, we recite the prayers of *Yizkor*, "Remembrance." Even as we are engaged in poignant self-judgment, hoping to be sealed for a future in the metaphoric Book of Life, we pause, look backward, and remember those who preceded us. At *Yizkor* we bring to mind the memories of our parents and grandparents, brothers and sisters, and friends, all those who touched our lives. *Yizkor Elohim nishmot yakirai*, we recite, "May God remember the souls of my loved ones."

Rabbi Jeffrey Marx of Santa Monica taught me, "We remember, not just for the sake of those who are dead, but for our own sake. To remember those who came before us is to know who we are." In remembering the past lies the key to the present and a path to the future. In remembering lies the secret of redemption. What then happens when one's memory begins to fail—when bits of data, elements of who one is, cannot easily be recalled? What happens when the obligation to remember can no longer be kept?

I recently acquired a new smartphone, that palm-sized telephone computer on which I store my address book, calendar, lists of birthdays and anniversaries, my to-do lists, and even a plethora of ideas for future sermons and projects. My wife says it is just a toy; for me it is my life. One evening, the data on the iPhone began to fade out. I could not access critical pieces of information. Before my eyes, I was losing the record of my past, even as I saw the hopes and dreams that I had stored about the future also fizzle out.

Fortunately, the memory loss was temporary. It is amazing how easily the data could be recalled from its permanent storage on our backup device. But what if . . . ? If losing a computer record of my past upset me so much, how would I feel if I truly began to lose my actual memory? And then I remembered Grandma Esther.

Tipped Off by Brownies

Grandma Esther was famous for delicious baked desserts. Her chocolate chip mandel bread was mouthwatering. Her upside-down cakes were sweetly tasty. But her brownies—so chewy—were the best.

Grandma's brownies were always perfectly square. We secretly joked that she must have measured each one with a ruler. I learned later that she did, in fact, use a ruler, and that every misshapen brownie was secreted away in her belly.

My father tells us that it was brownies that gave away the extent to which Alzheimer's disease had begun to claim Grandma's memory. One day, she frantically called her son, my father Kenny, asking him to come over quickly. Upon arrival he saw the problem: in the midst of baking brownies, Grandma's hand towel had become caught in the food processor. Some might have dismissed the incident as a technical problem; however, we knew better. Esther, a master baker who had made thousands of batches of brownies over her lifetime without a single mishap, had begun to lose her ability to bake her cakes.

Every family that has a member with Alzheimer's disease has its own "brownie incident," the moment that marked the family's descent into darkness. Denise Cooper, watching a similar tragedy play out as she cared for her loved one stricken with Alzheimer's disease, composed these beautiful words, titled "The Watcher:"[1]

> I watch you as you sleep, wondering if tomorrow will bring you
>   peace. I grieve for you.
> I watch you as you laugh, wondering if it will be the last. I
>   love you.
> I watch you as you speak, wondering if the words will come. I
>   am inspired.
> I watch you as you roam, wondering if you are looking for
>   home. I miss you too.
> I watch you as you walk, wondering how you bear the pain. I
>   hurt for you.
> I watch you as you sleep, wondering if tomorrow will bring you
>   peace. I mourn you.

Denise's words capture the worry, pain, wonder, and fear that accompany the reality of Alzheimer's disease. The Alzheimer's Association estimates that one in ten American families has a loved one with

Alzheimer's disease and that one in three adults knows someone with the disease. Many people struggling with this memory loss worry about eventually overwhelming their family caregivers as the disease progresses.

Caregivers have their own issues. Many are scared and overwhelmed. They describe feeling alone and disconnected from friends. Like many, they need assistance but are reluctant to ask. Needing a break from caregiving, they may not have anyone to relieve them. Experiencing stress, sometimes severe, they are looking for someone to listen.

Community and Family Help Remember

When a family is stricken with the plague of Alzheimer's disease, family members need help to experience God's love. People with Alzheimer's disease, their spouses, partners, children, and families can form a sacred community to assist each other as they traverse the inevitable darkness ahead. Yet so many do not know how to act, react, or respond. Friends and relatives may want to offer help but worry that they will say or do the wrong thing. Caregivers may desperately desire assistance but are uncomfortable sharing or foisting the burden of responsibility on others.

Al tifrosh . . . do not separate from the community. When the sense of alienation and aloneness is overwhelming, how can the family—as a community—respond? It takes a system of support to endure the unrelenting indignities and pain of Alzheimer's disease. A thoughtful and self-reflective family, or extended community, can create and reinforce a support system that validates the sadness and sense of loss, assist in the overwhelming responsibilities that arise, and spell the primary caregiving family member so he or she can find a little respite.

The caregiver and the patient both need us to listen. They need us to reach out. We need to make it a point as individuals and as a community to keep in touch by phone, to send cards, and to make extra portions of meals and drop them off for the caregiver. We can offer to stay with the person with Alzheimer's disease for a short period so that the family member can run errands, attend a support group, or catch a movie. We can visit and offer a shoulder to cry on or a sympathetic ear to listen. Moreover, we can spend time with the person with Alzheimer's disease and talk to him or her the way we would want someone to talk to us. The person may not be able to show it, but he or she will appreciate the visits.

Jerry Ham, a fifty-eight-year-old licensed practical nurse, stayed at home full-time for nearly six years to care 24/7 for his mother, who passed away from Alzheimer's disease in September 2001. His poem, "We Are Not a Machine,"[2] beautifully articulates the exhaustion and the often-overlooked needs of caregivers:

> We are the caregivers, but wait, there is more.
> So please, hear us out before closing the door.
> No we're not perfect, but we're doing our best.
> We just want to get some things off our chests.
>
> When was the last time you tried to come by,
> Or the last time you called, if only to say hi?
> Do you really realize just what we do here?
> And just how often we are driven to tears? . . .
>
> Even better, a visit from family and friends,
> To laugh, to talk, and smile once again.
> We must be honest, we don't want to demean.
> But please understand, we are not a machine.

The Role of the Synagogue

The Jewish community, especially synagogues, can provide important support and connections for families facing Alzheimer's disease.

At my former synagogue, Temple Beth Hillel in Valley Village, California, our Caring Community Task Force began a project wherein temple members reached out and called homebound members every week. On the list to receive a call was a longtime member who was stricken with Alzheimer's disease. A discussion ensued regarding whether he should be called, since he could not develop a relationship with the caller—which was an important aspect of the program—because he would not remember the call. Nevertheless, members of the task force decided to include him because the mitzvah, the obligation, was to reach out and help. How the recipient internalized the overture was a separate issue. More importantly, the point was that for that moment of the call, the person with Alzheimer's disease, his family, and the whole congregation all knew that they were connected to one another. This connection exists *l'dor vador*, "from generation to generation," whether one remembers it or not.

In the midrash,[3] Rav Joseph teaches "that the second set of tablets of the Ten Commandments and the broken tablets [that Moses shattered upon discovering the Golden Calf] were both kept in the Holy Ark. From here we learn that a scholar who has involuntarily forgotten his learning should not be treated disdainfully." *Kal vachomer*, how much more so it is vital that our loved ones, those who like the broken tablets still retain their holiness, continue to be held closely by us, by their caregivers, and by God.

At my current synagogue, Congregation Or Ami in Calabasas, California, our Henaynu Caring Community Committee lifts the veil of silence that surrounds Alzheimer's disease. Our Center for Jewish Parenting offers workshops on dealing with aging parents that address specific challenges facing families with Alzheimer's disease. Our three-times-a-year phone bank ensures that all members receive calls. Both activities lead us to create connections between families facing Alzheimer's disease so that they can support each other within the congregational community. Each Shabbat, by including Alzheimer's disease among the concerns about which we ask when we sing the *Mi Shebeirach* prayer for healing, we further sensitize the community to its responsibility to see and respond to people struggling with it. Every other year, we hold a special Shabbat service honoring caregivers. Beyond the stated purpose of blessing those who give of themselves to care for others, the service serves to coax the caregiver out of the home—at least for an evening—and to again create connections between people living through this nightmare.

A teaching by Reb Nachman of Bratzlav, grandson of the Baal Shem Tov, that I have heard in many places and in many ways might be helpful. Reb Nachman tells the story of a village that was hit with a plague that would temporarily erase memories. The townspeople, fearful of the chaos to come, searched high and low for an antidote to the disease, but to no avail. Finally, their attention turned to how they would endure the plague. No one knew what to do. Suddenly, a man walked up to the massive boulder at the center of the village square, and wrote upon it the four Hebrew letters—*Yod-Hei-Vav-Hei*—of God's divine name. Curious, the villagers questioned his action.

The man responded, "That we will soon forget the past is unavoidable. How that will affect our present and future is unknown. The letters of God's name, which according to the Torah connect to the eternality of existence, will indicate to us that there once was something that was enduring and had meaning. Let these letters, expressing the sanctity of existence, anchor our present and future to the abiding nature of our existence. Let God's eternal love transcend our momentary forgetfulness." As family, friends, and congregational community, we extend God's love to those who forget how to receive it.

Losing Grandma Esther

I have a vivid memory of Grandma Esther from years before Alzheimer's disease appeared in her life, showing off collages of pictures on the wall between the kitchen and her bedroom. They were a gift from her children, on Eddie and Esther's twenty-fifth anniversary. Grandma would delight in telling stories about each photo. There is a much younger, svelte Esther with a dapper Eddie, photographed back when they were "keeping company," Grandma's way of talking about dating. There is Bubbe and Papa, her parents. He was a carpenter, she a seamstress and then a mother of four. There are aunts and uncles, nieces and nephews, cousins, and us. Each picture, mostly in black and white, told a story. Esther, back then, remembered and could tell stories about each one.

But as Alzheimer's disease ravaged her mind, she began forgetting. Still, she lived on, slowly losing those parts of herself that made her who she was: her desire to cook, her ability to feed herself, her memory of loved ones, and her concern for how she looked. Like many family members of Alzheimer's disease patients, her son Kenny, my dad, would depart from his visits with her feeling frustrated. "Don't you remember, Ma? When we did this or that?" Impatience masked the incredible sadness of losing a loved one even as she lived on. Toward the end, Esther's memories gave way to fantasies—Dad became Eddie, her late husband—until her son's despair finally replaced his initial frustration.

When Death Finally—Blessedly—Arrives

Grandma Esther spent her last days at a nursing home on Cape Cod, where she often sat in a wheelchair. Alzheimer's disease slowly eroded her mind and memories, until a swift but painful bout of pancreatic cancer blessedly took her from the community she could no longer remember.

Through the years, I have listened while many a family would exclaim, following the death of an Alzheimer's disease patient, that they have been mourning the loss for a long time. Having watched their loved ones wither away for months or years, most expect the formal mourning process, and the emotional roller coaster that accompanies it, to be abbreviated or more easily tolerated. Many family members are so relieved to no longer have to watch their loved one decline that they cannot believe the pain could be any worse. Later, I am told, they realize that the pain of watching a loved one lose their memory does not negate the pain of losing the loved one physically. In a sense, many families of Alzheimer's disease patients face a double round of mourning: first, as the loved one loses him- or herself, and later, when the physical death eclipses the loss of self.

A family and the larger Jewish community should remember that the mitzvah, or religious obligation, of *halvayat hameit*, accompanying our dead to their final resting place, does not end at the cemetery, but continues until the survivors can walk with some sense of confidence and strength into their new lives. Our tradition teaches that this consumes the better part of a year. The community should refrain from offering comments about how relieved the mourners must be that their beloved is finally at peace. And, the community serves its members by preparing to support the mourners of an Alzheimer's disease patient. We slowly, patiently, share stories from the loved ones' past and regularly invite the mourners to tell stories so we too can remember their loved ones.

Zachor—Remember

When memory deteriorates or ceases to function, when *zachor*, remembering the past, becomes difficult, one can still find and offer a sense of *shalom*, "wholeness," in the present. In the Shabbat prayer *Adon Olam*, we sing, *V'hu hayah, v'hu hoveh, v'hu yih'yeh b'tifarah*, "God was, God is, and God will be forever more." Judaism teaches that through God, the past, present, and future are all connected. When we say, *Sh'ma Yisrael, Adonai Eloheinu, Adonai Echad*, "Hear, O Israel, *Adonai* is our God, *Adonai* is One," we are connecting ourselves to the Creator, thereby recognizing that God's oneness transcends what we can remember in the past and what we can envision in the future.

Isn't that what a community—a family—of caring does? Where the person cannot remember for herself, we will remember with her and for her. We can reach out to show her that we remember her, who she was and who she is. We can ground her and her family in the *k'neset Yisrael*, the "community of Israel." We can be that beacon of light that provides a sense of safety and security, a sense of connectedness. We can replace lost memory with unending love.

Jerry Ham, an Alzheimer's disease caregiver, who has written many wonderful poems about caregiving, captured this notion beautifully in his poem "You Do It for Love." Jerry writes:[4]

> You give of your heart, your love and your life,
> To a grandparent, parent, husband or wife.
> So often you feel like there's nobody there,
> No one to talk to, no one who cares.
>
> Then late at night, you'll sit up and cry,
> "It all seems so hopeless, so why do I try?"
>
> "You do it for love, you know that is true.
> "This love that you have, will help see you through.
> "You are not alone, there's someone who'll share,
> "The burden you carry, I'll help you bear."
> Then in the darkness, a warmth you can feel,
>
> A soft gentle presence, you know it is real.
> As you drop off to sleep, (a voice) from above,
> Echoes the words . . . "You do it for love."

So that is what we do. When memory fails, we—the family, the community—let love take its place.

4

✦

Early Responses: Talking to Dementia with Its Own, New Language

Bonnie Ann Steinberg

One warm Sunday morning, I was meeting with a young couple planning their wedding. I turned on the air conditioner in my office, and we began discussing all the things that need to get talked about before a wedding. All of a sudden, one of the elders of our congregation came up the stairs. He was angry. Loudly complaining about the noise from the air conditioner, he berated us for using the office at this hour, disturbing his Sunday morning while he was trying to read the newspaper in peace on his terrace adjoining the temple office. One of my regulars at services, his was the outburst of a very frustrated man, perhaps mixed with the pleasure of being able to criticize the rabbi. We all knew this man—he had watched the bride grow up in the congregation and knew her parents well. His anger concerned and confused us. As rabbis, we do our jobs at all sorts of hours, yet we had disturbed the peace that he was seeking. His peace and his family's peace were soon further disturbed by the growing realization that he was in the beginning stages of dementia. His angry outburst was an early symptom.

The couple and I felt guilty as we continued our meeting; it was a parallel guilt to that we all feel as we realize we cannot help others while we watch their illness progress. Our concern is tinged with the vague anxiety that it might happen to any one of us, myself included: How will I know, how will it begin, how will I understand my own symptoms? Will I embarrass myself, and how will I get the care that I might need? How will my family and friends adapt?

The great ethical question of our aging society is how we understand and care for all kinds of disabled people. There are unique challenges involved in caring for people who cannot express themselves, who cannot explain their needs, and who cannot advocate for themselves. There are very unique problems in caring for our loved ones with dementia because they are beyond conversation. The normal understandings about interaction and communication just don't apply. *How do we talk with dementia?* The person with dementia will still need all of our love and compassion, understanding and patience, caregiving and company, but the communications coming from the person with dementia will be very hard to translate into common language.

Adjusting and learning to communicate with such a person takes much practice.

We can learn of this form of communication from our finest medieval Jewish sage, Rabbi Moses ben Maimon, known as Maimonides, or by his acronym, Rambam. Maimonides was not only our greatest Jewish thinker in Torah, Talmud, and Jewish law, but he also served as physician to the noble court and wrote treatises on medical practice and ethics. In a philosophical tractate called *Sefer HaMada*, "The Book of Knowledge," which served as the introduction to his *Mishneh Torah*, his code of Jewish law, Maimonides wrote, "A wise man does not shout and scream when he speaks, but talks gently with all people, and never raises his voice unduly. He gives everyone a friendly greeting. . . . If he finds that his words are helpful and heeded, he speaks; otherwise, he keeps quiet."[1] (Although Maimonides wrote using the male pronoun, "he," we understand in this chapter that his instructions applied to men and women equally.) From our sage we learn that speaking compassionately to every person—even the one who may not understand, even those who are developing cognitive impairments due to increasing dementia, or who are living with a different language, the language of dementia— is mandated by our tradition. Surely, it requires adjusting and learning, and patience, too. Just as Rambam counseled keeping quiet when speech would be unhelpful, so too restraint, patience, and forbearance are part of the art of talking to dementia.

Moreover, our sage added a subtle, additional pearl of wisdom: we note that Rambam directed his instruction to the *wise man*. A wise man or woman, we could surely assume, would commonly be speaking to a person of lesser wisdom, from which we may derive an ethical charge regarding speaking to dementia: we are not to desist from engaging with those of lesser capacities, even if communication is difficult. That the other is less than able or speaks in his or her own dementia-driven language, does not relieve us from the charge to engage in such communication.[2]

In some people, forgetting has its charms. My friend lives with the results of a traumatic brain injury sustained in an automobile accident. Her father is in the middle stages of Alzheimer's disease. My friend always had a great sense of humor. At dinner together one night, she said, "I am having such a good time, it's too bad I won't remember this tomorrow." Meanwhile, my friend's dad, a lover of ice cream, ate bowl after bowl, trying to mix it with his napkin, his body forgetting that he had eaten enough ice cream, forgetting that the white napkin was not part of the white ice cream. We let him have his pleasure. I knew that perhaps one day his body would not know how to eat, how to feel that pleasure. It put us in a good mood to have a good time together. The good time is still worth it even if we won't remember it.

After the little things—the shadow of a blank look, the new way of forgetting—the going gets rough. A friend walked in as her mother was trying to put her pants over her head. At first you try to manage it at home. You get someone to help during the day, and then you can't sleep at night, while your loved one awakens at any hour ready to go out, to work, to shop. You think that you should be able to handle it. But since you can no longer talk to the person in our normal language and you can't get your dear one to reply in our regular language, you are not only exhausted but confused. The one-way nature of the relationship, even when you do the right things and say the right things, yields unpredictable outcomes.

We remember the counsel of Rambam, that the wise person speaks gently with all people and gives each a friendly greeting. Perhaps Maimonides's admonition, though surely helpful and instructive to the wise person or fellow sage, is even more meaningful and prescient to the one who is talking to dementia. This truly entails a new language. But, even with a new language, the same ethical directives regarding the previous language still hold or become even more pronounced: to speak gently and give friendly greetings. Experience in speaking to babies or to pets proves that even when one, such as an infant or a dog, cannot cognitively comprehend the meaning of words or of language, they nevertheless can discern the emotion, mood, and attitude of the communication. Thus, Rambam's instruction of the friendly greeting especially speaks volumes in the new language of talking to dementia.

On Friday nights, my friends Max and Julia meet Max's mother at temple. Max's mother had a stroke a few years previously, leaving her with vascular dementia. She had earlier purchased long-term care insurance, which thankfully supports her in her home with a full-time series of aides. Max, Julia, and Max's sister manage the aides and live with the uncertainty that their mom is getting adequate care. After work late Friday afternoons, the aide brings Max's mom to temple; Max and Julia finish work and meet her in the same sanctuary seats every Friday. After temple they all go to their favorite Friday night restaurant. On holidays, mom is part of the celebrations and dinners. One can see that Jewish music, prayer, and ritual connect somewhere in her memory bank. After Shabbat services, she says, "That was a good service." And during the Passover seder, her eyes look bright.

Yet, for the first years, Max and Julia would try to correct their mom when she made a "mistake." Mom would say about her son, Max, with a loving but mistaken pride, "He's my husband." Or she would look with confusion at Julia and say, "Are you married? Do you have children?" In fact, Max looks exactly like his father. I can remember Max's father; he does look exactly like him. But Max and

Julia would try to explain, saying patiently, "No, Mom. Remember: Dad died, and this is Max, your son. And yes we are married, and these are your grandchildren." Max's mom would look at him and take it in somehow, but she was not convinced. She would repeat the same question, and Max and Julia would try to correct her, hoping that all she needed was a little reminder.

It took Max and Julia a while to understand that the language of dementia cannot be corrected. We cannot offer corrections and reminders. We have to understand that the communication is "other." Max's mother is remembering in her new way. Conversations and stories might come from some other dimension of the brain's new understanding. If Julia and Max say, "Tell me about your husband," they might get a story. They cannot explain that Max is her son. That language just cannot be corrected.

If anything can reach inside this new brain and its new language, it is the very old and emotive language of music. If Jewish music was part of a person's memory bank, then often music will still connect. I have sung *Shalom Aleichem, Adon Olam, Ein Keloheinu,* Chanukah songs, "Jerusalem of Gold," and countless other songs with people with dementia. They may not recognize their own family members, but very often they can sing along.

Thus, we cannot speak to dementia, and we cannot fix it by giving the person the right information. We cannot have a logical conversation with someone who has dementia, yet we need to acknowledge their words as reflecting their reality. We need to use their words to access that reality, to pursue their thought as they present it; we need to let their words lead us into their reality. We cannot fix their memories or correct their information by giving the person the right information. We can only learn to manage each hour, mourning the loss of the mind that once drove the body and organized its speech, trying to figure out how to read this new form of communication coming from this person with dementia. We must seek to communicate our love to someone who cannot understand the old forms of communication. Ironically, this person now needs to receive even more communication and more caring than one person can give.

Calibrating this new, uneasy equilibrium also was addressed by Maimonides, though not directly in reference to Alzheimer's disease or to dementia. In another philosophical treatise, called *Sh'monah P'rakim: A Treatise on the Soul*, the Rambam wrote about sickness of the soul and its imbalances. Referring to persons whose behavior went to extremes and missed the balanced middle way, which, as an Aristotelian philosopher, Rambam strongly advocated, Maimonides wrote, "We referred to this when we spoke of equilibrium—neither adding nor subtracting. . . . One should not go to either extreme except as a matter of medicine. . . . Should someone know that one part of one's body is weak, one should constantly take care of it . . . and try to improve it or at least not allow it to be further weakened."[3] Although Rambam was not directly addressing those with dementia, he was concerned with balance and imbalance, and he promoted returning to such a balance, if at all possible. For those with Alzheimer's disease or dementia, returning to any such previous plateau of balance cannot be expected, yet Rambam's charge to "not allow it to be further weakened" offers an encouraging mandate. Even if we know that the dementia will steadily decline, Rambam nevertheless demands intervention or engagement, at the very least to sustain the individual at various plateaus or equilibriums along the progression of the disease. His charge, therefore, was toward arresting illness before it reaches extremes. For the person with Alzheimer's disease, we can derive from Rambam the instruction to seek and embrace the plateaus along the way.

People are very reluctant to place their loved ones into nursing homes. I work in one of the largest not-for-profit nursing homes in New York State. I cannot rightfully claim that the nursing home is perfect, but in the caring, well-managed nursing home, there is a large community of diverse staff to share the complex tasks, or shoulder the majority of those tasks with families and significant others as we work to care for people with dementia. Eventually, a family, spouse, or significant other cannot provide this care alone.

For instance, Richard was a very elegant, charming, and intelligent person. His wife wanted a few good years of retirement with him, and some great trips and dinners out with friends, but dementia set in. She cared for him at home for as long as she could, and then she reluctantly placed him in our nursing home. A few years passed and she adjusted to the routines of visiting and trying to feel that she could have a life without him, and not feeling too upset and guilty when imperfect things happened at the nursing home. Eventually, Richard no longer really recognized her or their children. She would bring him to religious services and music programs, sometimes wondering if it was worth it any longer. Yet, after Rosh HaShanah services, Richard said, "More, more." He had not spoken a coherent word in a few years. Sometimes, during a music event, Richard's wife could sense him taking the music in, even when he could not understand anything that was spoken to him otherwise.

A familiar biblical text, which perhaps might have resonated with Richard, is the famous injunction "Love your neighbor as yourself" (Leviticus 19:18). Maimonides addressed this text in his *Sefer HaMada*, his introduction to his code of Jewish law, adding his commentary, "Hence, we must speak of him in terms of praise. . . . 'Whoever glorifies himself by humiliating someone else has no share in the future world' (Jerusalem Talmud, *Chagigah* 2:1)."[4] Strikingly, as Rambam contrasted the experience of treating another person with care and not humiliating the other, we learn that the biblical command is not merely to love another as *oneself*, but to love the other as one who is *different* from oneself! It is easy to love or revere a person who is the same as or greater than oneself, but it is a challenge to love the one who is lesser or different. This, Rambam argues, is the ethic behind the famous biblical command.

Mr. Cohen seems alert when I walk into the room, his yarmulke tipping forward on his forehead. He is in bed, sitting up. His wife sits nearby; she is young-looking for eighty-three, slim, with her makeup on, jeans, and a lacy shirt. She stands to greet me, and while we talk, she is both energetic and tired. She is glad that I came. She wants to talk about what is transpiring with her husband. She could still care for her husband at home until a few months earlier, when he fell and it was too difficult for her to raise him. He fell a second time, and this time she really needed help. It was time to consider nursing home care. While her husband was recovering from his broken hip, Mrs. Cohen made a difficult discovery: it was easier to sleep at night knowing that her husband was in a safer place. She worried and felt guilty; shouldn't she be able to take care of him at home? He wasn't that sick. Mrs. Cohen needed to talk. Occasionally her husband would try to enter the conversation, and it was clear that he was in the early stages of dementia. He said what he wanted, but she thought that he needed correction. He got sequences of events wrong, and she corrected him. He called me the rebbetzin, and she corrected him. She apologized for his rudeness. He tried to reenter the conversation, and she became frustrated with his misunderstandings and his mistakes, and his words didn't make sense to her. She was frustrated. "You can see what I am dealing with," she explained to me. Normal communication was absent; it was the new language of dementia speaking.

None of us can talk our normal, cognitively based language to dementia. We need to adjust and find new balances, as Rambam taught. We need to pick up new signals and adapt to new ways of communicating. Our job is to sing, to accompany, to present Jewish ritual when rituals can give context or comfort, and to give support to the family and staff, because they—the music, accompanying, the ritual, the support—become the new symbols and mechanisms in this new language of talking with dementia. Our job is to mourn the loss of the mind that used to inform the body according to our normal logic. The body is still there, while the brain or mind increasingly miscommunicates to the body, which still needs food, clothing, washing, and care. Yet, the mind is still there in a new form. It still needs peace and comfort and love.

People with dementia need us to remember who they were when they could still communicate in our way. Those persons need us to learn to communicate in their new language. Our job is to imagine that we are the person with dementia and to think about how we would like to be treated. Love your neighbor as yourself.

5

꙳

Questions of Legal Competency

ELLIOT N. DORFF

I would imagine that virtually everyone reading this book has witnessed at least one person who suffered with Alzheimer's disease. I have known several, but the one who immediately comes to mind is Rabbi Max Vorspan, who was among the founders of the university where I work. Max wrote the authoritative book on the history of the Jews of Los Angeles, and for many years he produced and hosted a television program on current affairs. He was a bright, effervescent person, with sparkling eyes and unbelievable creativity and energy. The story that always comes to mind when I think of him was a particular graduation day, when everything was going wrong: the air conditioning was not working, the person who received an honorary degree who was supposed to speak for three minutes spoke for fifteen, and the choir that was supposed to sing two songs sang five. Then it was Max's turn to speak as the designated commencement speaker. I remember thinking to myself that if I were he, I would say to the audience, "You really do not want to hear this," and sit down. Instead, in ten minutes he completely changed the mood in the room, such that nobody remembered what had happened earlier. He was simply scintillating. And then he was diagnosed with Alzheimer's, and it was absolutely excruciating to watch his mind deteriorate—this smart, funny, energetic, and challenging man no longer able to recognize any of his family or friends or string words into a sentence. It is to Max—and to all those who, like him, have been devastated by this disease, as well as their caregivers—that I dedicate this essay.

Treating the Body and the Mind

If it was difficult to discover effective medications for the body before the twentieth century, it was all the more difficult to treat illnesses of the mind. The Bible describes in detail the paranoid psychopathia and perhaps the epilepsy of King Saul, and others in the Bible and Talmud suffer from visual and auditory hallucinations, insanity, and "possession by demons or spirits."[1] Biblical prophets experienced trances and ecstasies. In antiquity, Jews interpreted such phenomena positively, as proof of divine contact. The people who babbled incoherently were thus not described and denounced as insane; they were rather held in esteem as prophets.

The later tradition, though, treated reports of such experiences negatively, as signs of illness. Jews then sought to exorcise the ghosts (*sheidim*) or furies (*dybbuks*) that caused them. They often used music in an attempt to seduce demons to leave the minds of the insane and thereby calm and cure them.

In modern times, of course, we have learned to diagnose and distinguish many mental illnesses, and researchers have developed therapies far more effective than those used in ancient, medieval, or early modern times to diminish their deleterious effects. Indeed, people suffering from some of those diseases can now live fulfilling lives and function in society. Unfortunately, even though scientists have made headway in diagnosing Alzheimer's, they have not yet been able to prevent or cure it. This has posed a challenge not only to medical research, but also to those concerned with Jewish law, for it raises questions of legal competency.

Defining Insanity

It should be noted that in the Jewish tradition there is no term for Alzheimer's disease per se. Rather, there is the category of *sh'tut*, "insanity," and, as we shall see, the category of someone who is sometimes clearheaded and sometimes not. Scholars and bioethicists use these categories as most relevant to the cognitive loss associated with Alzheimer's disease in order to apply Jewish law to both the later and earlier stages of the condition.

Because insanity had legal implications, described below, the Rabbis tried to define it as specifically as possible:

> Our Rabbis taught: Who is deemed insane? He who goes out alone at night, and he who spends the night in a cemetery, and he who tears his garments. It was taught: Rabbi Huna said, "He must do all of them [to be considered insane]." Rabbi Yochanan said, "Even if [he does only] one of them." It was taught: Who is deemed insane? One who destroys everything given to him.[2]

Maimonides correctly notes that the behaviors listed in the Talmudic source quoted above are to be construed as symptoms, not as an exhaustive definition of insanity.[3] In line with this, Moshe Halevi Spero, a contemporary Orthodox psychologist, suggests specific criteria for determining mental disorders—rather than just examples of what an insane person might do—for purposes of legal excuse in Jewish law. "Generally speaking," he says, "*shtus* (or, in the Sephardic pronunciation, *sh'tut*, meaning 'mental incompetence' or 'insanity') might denote one who has lost the ability to reason or make reality-based judgments. *Shtus* may also signify the loss of emotional control."[4]

Early Attempts to Address the Legal Issues Posed by Insanity

A diagnosis of insanity had many legal implications in Jewish law. When the degree of mental incompetence warranted it, the Rabbis of the Mishnah and Talmud exempted the insane from responsibility in both ritual and civil law. At the same time, they made the insane ineligible for certain legal roles (for example, serving as another person's legal agent).[5] They also sought to define the exact degree and scope of legal responsibility of someone who did not have full free will as a result of his or her own decisions, as, for example, those under the influence of alcohol or drugs.[6]

The general approach in Jewish sources was to disenfranchise the mentally ill as little as possible. So, for example, after the bands of prophets during biblical times,[7] we do not hear of Jewish communities isolating the mentally ill.

Moreover, the Rabbis distinguished between those times when a person was apparently sane, and therefore legally capable, and those times in which she or he was not.[8] This was especially of interest in determining when a man was mentally competent to instruct his agent to issue a writ of divorce (a *get*) to his wife, for in classical Jewish law only the man may initiate a divorce. The Talmud recognizes that it may be the case that *itim halim, itim shoteh* (sometimes he is of sound mind, and sometimes he is insane), and it decreed that when a person was sane, he was sane for all legal purposes, and when he was insane, he was insane for all legal purposes.[9] Only a person whose mind is permanently damaged is legally categorized as insane for all his or her actions.[10] Therefore, the trick was to determine when a person was of sound mind so that he had the legal competence to authorize the issuance of a *get* to his wife.[11] The same concern applied to legal competency to betroth,[12] and it also applied to transact a sale:[13] if one could determine that the person was sane when the betrothal or sale occurred, then the betrothal or sale was valid, but otherwise it was not.[14] Ritual acts and leading prayer must also be done by mentally competent people, and thus the Talmud discusses the issue of determining whether the slaughterer was sane or not with regard to killing the paschal lamb.[15]

Most importantly, insane people cannot be held criminally responsible for their acts.[16] Thus the Mishnah says, "It is a bad thing to strike a deaf-mute, a mentally defective person, or a minor, for one who injures any one of them is liable, but if any one of them wounds someone else, he is not liable."[17] Even the unconsciousness of sleep constitutes a legal excuse of duress with regard to criminal acts, for sleeping people lack criminal (or any other) intent; unlike insane people, however, sleeping people are liable for any civil damages they cause.[18] People who suffer from transient attacks of insanity, such as epileptics and people in the early stages of Alzheimer's, are criminally responsible only for acts committed during lucid periods.[19] Because the insane are devoid not only of reason but also of will, any sexual offenses they commit are deemed to have been committed unwillfully, and therefore such people are exempt from the criminal penalties associated with such acts for sane people.[20]

Precisely because sanity is a critical factor in establishing both legal competence and legal liability, contemporary rabbinic authorities are keenly interested in the progress of psychology as a science to help determine when a person is sane and when not.

Mental Illness as a Disease

Probably the most important legal step in the history of Jewish law with regard to mental illness has been its classification as an illness rather than a moral fault. The Talmud asserts that virtually all obligations and prohibitions may be set aside to save a person's physical life (*pikuach nefesh*).[21] It also permitted lighting a candle in violation of the Sabbath rules for a woman in labor in order to spare her psychic anguish.[22] Citing that precedent, Nachmanides (thirteenth century) included mental illness in the category of "saving one's life" (*pikuach nefesh*), so that the same exemptions from the law as normally practiced would apply in emergency situations to saving a person's mental health.[23] This argument is used by many rabbis in modern times to justify abortion on the grounds of mental health, not as a retroactive form of birth control but when the mother will suffer major mental anguish if she delivers the child.[24] It can also be used to do what is necessary in order to save people with Alzheimer's from doing things that are harmful to themselves or others, either mentally or physically, even if it involves violating some of the ritual or moral laws of Judaism.

Because both physical and mental illnesses were usually incurable, the Jewish tradition sought to prevent disease. With regard to the body, many of the tradition's precautions actually worked to prevent the spread of disease. So, for example, the Torah already stipulates that a community must quarantine those who are sick to stop the spread of communicable diseases (Leviticus 13–14)—and quarantine was still the method in use in the 1950s in the United States to limit the spread of measles, mumps, chicken pox, and polio until vaccines were eventually developed for those diseases.

Similarly, because mental illness was likewise often incurable, the Jewish tradition sought to prevent it by offering advice for maintaining mental health, often suggesting the cultivation of specific personal characteristics and values. The biblical Book of Proverbs, with its counsel on living a virtuous life, provides an early instance of such advice. Perhaps the most famous example in Rabbinic literature is Ethics of the Fathers (*Pirkei Avot*), a tractate of the Mishnah (edited ca. 200 CE) that is read every Shabbat afternoon during the weeks between Passover and Shavuot, which similarly expounds on how to live righteously. A thousand years later Maimonides included in his law code a section on personality traits, *Hilchot Dei-ot*, in which he embraced the Aristotelian golden mean as the proper guideline for human behavior. He suggested that one who was very calm, for example, should try to go to the other extreme in order to maintain a balance of spirit.[25] Jews in Medieval Spain also produced important psychological-ethical handbooks, including *Chovot HaL'vavot* (*Duties of the Heart*) by Bachya ibn Pakuda (eleventh century), *Sefer HaChinuch* (*Book of Education*) attributed to Aaron HaLevi of Barcelona (thirteenth century), and *Kad HaKemach* (*Measure of Flour*) by Bachya ben Asher (thirteenth century). In the eighteenth century, the Italian Kabbalist Moses Chayim Luzzato wrote the ethical tract *M'silat Y'sharim* (*The Path of the Upright*).[26] In the nineteenth and twentieth centuries, the Musar movement spread through some Orthodox communities of Eastern Europe, seeking to balance the heavy emphasis on study of texts and intellectual analysis that was common in traditional seminaries with materials and meetings devoted to moral and spiritual development, resembling in some ways modern group therapy sessions.

In such ways, Jews sought to prevent or cure mental illness. However primitive their understanding of it was, Jews saw it not as something for which one should repent or be punished, but rather as an illness we must seek to prevent or cure as part of our general obligation to heal. This prepared the way for Sigmund Freud and many other Jews to develop and practice the modern medical forms of psychological care.

The Legal Duty to Avoid and Cure Disease

The Jewish tradition asserts that God owns us: "Mark, the heavens to their uttermost reaches belong to *Adonai* your God, the earth and all that is on it!" (Deuteronomy 10:14); "The earth is *Adonai*'s and all that it holds, the world and all its inhabitants" (Psalm 24:1). As a result, each of us has a fiduciary obligation to God to take care of ourselves, for we are, as it were, merely renting God's body during our lease on life. With regard to our physical bodies, this has meant that we must take precautions to avoid disease, including proper diet, exercise, hygiene, and sleep, and we must avoid behaviors that would injure our bodies, such as smoking, drug or alcohol abuse, and obesity. We must also be vaccinated—and vaccinate our children—for the many diseases that we can avoid in that way. Clinical medicine that provides these preventive measures, and remedies and research into creating new vaccines or cures for diseases, are both prized activities in the Jewish tradition precisely because they aid us in fulfilling our fiduciary responsibilities to God.

Furthermore, from the Torah to contemporary times, almost all of our sources assert that we have free will and therefore are responsible for what we do. Thus, although Judaism permits alcohol consumption, Jews are forbidden to put themselves into a situation where they knowingly will lack mental capacity—that is, getting drunk. If they do become inebriated, they are fully responsible in Jewish law for what they do in that state.[27] Moreover, those who aid and abet their drunkenness and/

or fail to keep them from engaging in dangerous behavior while drunk "strengthen the hands of those who commit a sin" (*achzekai* [or *machazikin*] *y'dai ovrei aveirah*).[28] This also violates Jewish law, even though the drunk person, and not the aide, is held legally responsible for what he does while drunk.

Judaism treats mental illness in the same way. At this moment in time, medications to prevent Alzheimer's disease and therapies to cure it do not exist. When they do—hopefully in the near future—Jews would be required to avail themselves of those measures to avoid or cure their mental disease, just as much as we have the duty to take the steps necessary to avoid or cure physical diseases. This is already the case for those with propensities for alcoholism, drug abuse, obesity, or smoking: Jews with any of those propensities have the legal duty to seek help to overcome or avoid them, just as people with diabetes must take insulin and monitor their sugar intake, people with asthma must use their preventive inhalers, and people with high blood pressure or cholesterol must take steps to lower those conditions.

Moreover, if, at such a time when preventive measures are available, Jews with early-onset Alzheimer's do not take the steps then available to avoid or cure their disease, they will be fully liable in Jewish law for whatever they do. Their caregivers who fail to help them in these ways will have failed in their duty to care for their loved one or patient and may even be seen as abetting any dangerous act they do to harm themselves or others.

We obviously, and painfully, are not at that stage yet. At present, we can only provide palliative and psychological support to those with this terrible disease. Those who have Alzheimer's in the early stages would be fully legally competent when they are in their "clear" moments and not legally competent when they lack mental clarity—a case exactly like the Talmud's *itim halim, itim shoteh*, "sometimes of sound mind and sometimes insane." As the disease progresses, the person will eventually be judged insane (*shoteh*), at which point he is exempt from any duties and from any liability, and he is legally incapable of performing any function for which legal sanity is required.

The Inherent Ambiguity in Judging
the Stages of the Disease

How do we know when that stage has been reached? Caregivers—
and, frankly, physicians—yearn for clear, objective criteria to make
that determination so that they do not have to depend on their own
judgment. Relatives fear that their understanding of the state of the
disease in a particular person may be clouded by their own exhaustion in caring for a loved one with Alzheimer's and their desire to end
at least the intensity of that care once the person cannot recognize
anyone any longer. Conversely, they may feel guilty if they distance
themselves from the care of their loved one too prematurely. At least
if they knew on objective grounds that their loved one was beyond the
stage of mental awareness and sanity, they could rest assured that it
was not just their intuition that such was so. Physicians wish that their
science and art could give them the objectivity that their patients and
their families seek from them—and that they could treat their patients
with objective tests that demonstrate that their diagnosis of the state of
the disease in a given person at a given time is correct. Unfortunately,
such tests are still not available to determine the stages of dementia.

As readers of this chapter have seen, the Talmud recognized long
ago that *itim halim, itim shoteh*, people with illnesses like Alzheimer's,
will mentally decline gradually over time, such that there is a period in
which people are sometimes clearheaded and sometimes not so, before
they reach the stage where they no longer have any reality testing or
memory whatsoever. That fact, which is still the case today, should
comfort us all in knowing that ambiguity is inherent in these situations. This means that all we can reasonably expect of ourselves and
our physicians is our best efforts to provide people with Alzheimer's
disease their due care, respect, and safety.

I have had many decades of dealing with issues that people face
at the end of life, and there is none more excruciating for caregivers than to watch the gradual deterioration that Alzheimer's disease
brings. Physical causes of death are often painful and rightfully evoke
our compassion, sympathy, and empathy, but when the mind goes, we

have a sense that the person is no longer there. The fact that the person him- or herself senses what is occurring in the early stages of the disease, the fear that that engenders, and the terrible dehumanization that occurs as the person loses all sense of reality are really hard to watch—especially when, as in Rabbi Max Vorspan's case, the person used to be really bright, intellectually alive, creative, and funny. We clearly need to support further research into this disease to seek therapies to prevent or cure it; but in the meantime, we need to provide the company that all people need for as long as those with Alzheimer's sense that someone cares about them, to say nothing of the medical ministrations and safety precautions that they need even after that stage. We then need to remember Alzheimer's patients as they were before the disease took its toll, for the ultimate way to honor them is to recall them as they were during most of their lives, before the disease struck. And if we stuck by them for as long as it seemed to make a difference to them, we have done all that we could possibly do, and we have carried out God's mandate to care even when we cannot cure.

6

⟿

Shining Through: Being a Daughter When Mom Is Changing

Ellen Dreskin

A young child walking home from synagogue with her mother says, "Mommy, may I ask you a question about the rabbi's sermon?"

"Of course, dear," replies her mother.

"Didn't the rabbi say that God was bigger than everyone?" asks the little girl.

"Yes, dear," replies the mother.

"But Mommy," continues the daughter, "didn't the rabbi also say that God is inside each and every one of us?" The mother thinks for a moment.

"Yes, dear, the rabbi also said that God is inside each and every one of us."

"Well," asks the little girl, "Here's what I don't understand. If God is bigger than all of us, and God is inside each of us, then isn't God bound to shine through?"

As my mother progresses through the various stages of Alzheimer's and that which was her life story is preserved only in scrapbooks and the stories that my siblings and I tell, I am constantly amazed at the holy spark of my mother's essence that still shines through. Since her diagnosis, my mother has survived the loss of almost all of her short-term memory, with her long-term memory not far behind, as well as a broken hip and arm from which she made a remarkable recovery, my father's death, and many other challenges. Yet, she remains, at her core, my mother, shining through.

Torah uses two different verbs, "honor" and "revere," when addressing the relationship between parent and child. Exodus 20:12, from the Ten Commandments, states, "Honor [*kabeid*] your father and your mother, that you may long endure on the land that *Adonai* your God is assigning to you." Leviticus 19:3, from the Holiness Code, com-mands, "You shall each revere [*tira-u*] your mother and father, and keep My Sabbaths: I *Adonai* am your God." What is the difference between honor and reverence? Does one take precedence over the other? And how do these obligations from child to parent change as one's parents age and their mental and physical faculties diminish?

In the Talmud, our early code of Jewish law, our Rabbis taught:

> What is fear/reverence, and what is honor? "Reverence" means that he [the son] must neither stand in his [the father's] place nor sit in his place, nor contradict his words, nor tip the scales against him. "Honor" means that he must give him food and drink, clothe and cover him, lead him in and out." (Babylonian Talmud, *Kiddushin* 31b–32a)

In my mother's house, the two verbs and their respective obligations went very much together.

My mother, Iris Helene (Bennett) Siegel, was born in October 1921. She had been married to my father for just over sixty years when he passed away in April of 2009. My parents raised three very indepen-dent children; each of us left home immediately after college and now reside in Colorado, Pennsylvania, and New York. My parents were quite vocal about their desire that at least one of us would return to settle in our hometown of Houston, and yet I know that it makes my mother proud that each of us had the strength and self-confidence to strike out on our own and pursue our dreams.

My mother is blind, having been diagnosed at an early age with retinitis pigmentosa. This disease, which manifests as night blindness, loss of peripheral vision, and, in my mother's case, eventual total blindness, is a major part of who my mother is and what it has meant to be her daughter.

It has never been possible for me to say that my mother "suffers from" or "is a victim of" retinitis pigmentosa. While she never had a driver's license and all of her books and magazines arrived on reel-to-reel or cassette tapes from Lighthouse for the Blind, I rarely saw the disease get in her way. She always moved confidently about our house, entertained guests, cooked meals, and loved to go out to restaurants and movies, and especially to musical events. With the aid of contact lenses, glasses, and her magnifying glass, she experimented with new recipes, played bridge with friends, and even transcribed textbooks for the Braille Institute. My mother was well-read, listened to the news on radio and TV every day, and had no trouble holding up her end of a conversation.

The Talmudic definition of "honor" as leading a parent in and out is particularly germane to my upbringing. It never struck me as odd that my mother always had company wherever she went. At the grocery store, my mother would have me read the shopping list aloud to her (a list that she had written contrary to the lines on the paper, and often with words inscribed on top of each other), and then she would supervise my placing the items in the basket. As if she had maps of the grocery store in her head, she would memorize exactly where our favorite items could be found in each aisle. Thanks to her excellent memory of street names, as well as her sense of direction and her childhood knowledge of Houston's geography, she often would be able to give friends detailed driving directions from one place to another. She never entertained the idea of a guide dog or a cane, insisting rather that she was perfectly capable of getting along without either one.

Throughout my childhood and adolescence, each time we left the house or the car, my dad would say, as if he knew the Talmud's instruction, "Someone grab Mom." And someone always did. There was no opportunity in my upbringing for that awkward adolescent stage of not wanting to be seen in public with my mother. Not only was I often in the company of my mother, but I was bound to have her on my arm. When someone approached her at a party or began speaking at a meeting, my mother was never shy about her blindness. She was very clear. "I'm sorry. I can't see. Who is speaking, please?" Her friends would always begin face-to-face conversations as if they were talking on the phone: "Hi Iris, it's Pat." And, there were numerous voices that my mother recognized in an instant, without any prompt or introduction. I marveled at her capacity to process and store so much information that most of us receive only visually.

Perhaps because she knew that she was often at the mercy of friends and strangers alike, my mother was always considerate, warm, and appreciative. She still is. It is part of her core that continues to shine through. I continue to learn from her how to transform what others might see as a severe disability into an opportunity to accept one's shortcomings or lack of experience or knowledge with honesty, grace, and charm. It is her default setting.

My family is fortunate that my father ensured that finances would be available should supplementary care become necessary. "Reverence," in the Talmudic sense, is maintained. Thanks to the tireless efforts of my sister and the boundless love and compassion of my mother's two main caregivers, Alicia and Deborah, my mother's physical needs have been more than met. My mother is still able to live in the same house that she has occupied since 1961. While she does not literally remember where she is most of the time, we know that there is a sense of familiarity in the rooms, voices, meals, and routines of the place and the people within it. Years ago, we contemplated moving my parents closer to one of their children so visits could be more frequent and less expensive, but that is no longer a viable option. At this point, honoring and revering my mother means allowing her to live within a recognizable routine, with minimum disruption, much music, and large doses of laughter. For the most part, we do not correct her when she is mistaken about events or conversations and are happy to follow her thoughts and ideas wherever they might go.

As Alzheimer's disease frees my mother from the demands of the daily clock, and her loss of vision liberates her even from realizing the difference between day and night, we honor and revere her in some perhaps more unorthodox ways. She awakens when she pleases, wears whatever she likes, eats when she is hungry, and rests whenever she feels it necessary or desirable. From time to time, my mother sleeps till noon, or eats the equivalent of breakfast, lunch, and dinner within ninety minutes of each other, or stays up till midnight watching old movies on TV. Because demands on her are few and because even her movement from one room to another is often accompanied by Ella Fitzgerald CDs and her caregiver's unique, rhythmical dance steps and harmonies, she is usually happy, open to suggestion, inquisitive without being fearful, and commonly able to laugh at her own confusion. When I call from New York and she seems troubled that she cannot remember where she is, I remind her that she is at her home in Houston. "How do you know?" she asks me. "Because that's where I called you!" I reply. It always gets a laugh.

Approximately five years ago, when my mother's memory capacity in a conversation was about ten to fifteen minutes, we engaged in philosophical discussions regarding one of the most important choices in my life: my decision to be a cantor. One Sunday morning when the two of us were alone together, my mother began, "Help me to understand. What is it about Judaism that is so compelling, so attractive to you?"

I offered a very descriptive shpiel about God and liturgy and social justice and the wonderful lessons that Judaism has to teach the world. When I took a breath at the end of fifteen minutes or so, my mother said, "I see. But what is it about Judaism that is so compelling, so attractive to you?"

I responded, "I just told you."

"I forget what you said," she replied. "Tell me again."

So I began again, this time with a little less verbiage, but also with a little more attitude. When I was done, my mother asked the same question, yet again. I responded, again, more succinctly. Inside my head, of course, I was increasingly frustrated that my mother was asking me the same question over and over again. And then I had a realization. My mother actually was not asking me the same question over and over again. She was asking a new question, from her point of view, every time. I was the one who was choosing to see each instance in the same way. I decided then to honor her and her questions with more deliberate answers. When I finally broke through my personal wall of frustration, I was able to enjoy my mother's company and her question, which came from a genuinely honest desire to understand. We spoke for nearly two hours, and by the time we were done, I had markedly refined my response to her inquiry regarding what was so compelling about Judaism, namely, gratitude and responsibility.

Reverence for the unwitting wisdom from my mother that is still able to shine through often reminds me of the passage from the morning liturgy, describing God as *ham'chadeish b'chol yom tamid ma'aseih v'reishit*, "the One who constantly renews the act of Creation each day." This prayer, called *Yotzeir Or*, praises God for periods of light, yet does so without overtly mentioning any direct light source, such as the sun or the moon. As well, it acknowledges God as the Maker of *shalom*, which I interpret as the state of complete balance over the course of lifetimes and universes: good, bad, light, dark, everything that exists in the world, along with its complete opposite. The prayer continues, "The land and all who dwell here are enlightened with great mercy." Finally, *Yotzeir Or* acknowledges that Creation occurs anew every moment of every day. The unraveling of my mother's memory and the inevitable frustration that comes with that loss have taught me a great lesson about making room for this constant process of re-Creation. My mother treats every mundane moment as something new. She is pleasantly surprised each time by the answer to a question that she has asked repeatedly. In the spirit of the *Yotzeir Or*, I have tried, as her daughter, to spend minimal time mourning the loss of who my mother used to be, and more time appreciating and honoring the spark that continues to shine through.

The gratitude and responsibility that shape my Jewish worldview also frame my relationship to my mother. These are my expressions of *kavod*/honor and *yirah*/reverence. I am extremely grateful that my mother makes it so easy to love her. I am ever more aware of all that my mother has given and continues to give, even at this stage of our lives. She continues to model grace, charm, and strength under very confusing circumstances. Even as emotional outbursts occur, or as she frequently obsesses on a single idea from a casual conversation, these moments may still be calmed with soothing words and lots of hugs. I know that it will not always be this way, and I am filled with gratitude for the blessings that my family has experienced thus far.

And I am still filled with reverence and respect for my mother as she is today. Even as she loses memories—the stories that she told herself and the ways she understood the experiences of her life—I am in awe of the holy spark that remains. She is, for the time being, optimistic, resilient, warm, and totally herself at her very core. She is no longer burdened by human drama, disappointments of the past, social obligations, or other people's preconceived notions of how she ought to behave. My mother's memory loss helps me to understand that our lives are shaped almost entirely by our memories, the stories that we tell ourselves, and the garments in which we clothe our individual experiences. All of that has been taken from my mother. And, having passed the frustration with her memory loss—that stage has come and gone—she simply marches to her own (jazz) drummer. Similarly, I continue to honor my mother by letting go of my old notions, my old stories, and any remaining baggage that clutters our relationship, and accepting each new stage as it comes.

Despite how dementia is changing my mother, it is amazing to me how she remains so much herself. Torah commands us "not to oppress the stranger, for you know the soul of the stranger" (Exodus 23:9). When my mother acts "strangely," it is usually because pressure has been applied—to her routine, to her memory, to her ability to function in unfamiliar circumstances. Our job now is to honor and revere her by relieving pressure. We know her soul. It is still there, undiminished.

There is an old Jewish folktale that relates a conversation that God had with the mythic angels before the creation of humankind. God wished to actively engage with the world and humanity, to somehow infuse the physical world with the Divine Presence. The angels objected: "Those humans beings will ruin it! If you insist on infusing the world with your divine spark, then at least hide it in a place where human beings will not be able to find it and corrupt it with their free will, selfish musings, and machinations." One angel suggested that God's spark should be hidden at the top of the highest mountain. Another advocated hiding it in the depths of the ocean.

God, however, knew better. "I shall place my holy spark at the core of the soul of each and every human being," said God. "That's the last place that they will ever look."

Yes, Alzheimer's disease has stolen much of my mother's life. But when we look to the core of her soul, what remains is her basic character, her resilience, her optimistic spirit, the Texas charm that has always been my mother, shining through.

Thank You, Source of Sources, for the spark that is my mother and for the joy that she is still able to wring from each puzzling moment. Thank You for compassionate and competent caregivers, for diligent and loving siblings, and for circumstances that allow my mother to be honored and revered as is her right. Thank You for teaching me, through my mother's life, that each and every moment, even those riddled with Alzheimer's disease, carries equal potential for surprise, wonder, and insight. And thank You, regardless of what the future brings, for continually allowing me to learn from this experience. Finally, thank You for the grace with which my mother sheds her past, allowing us the capacity to lovingly accept the holy spark that remains in every single moment.

7

❧

Dementia: As Seen by a Neurologist

RHONNA SHATZ

Like the Ark built by the ancient Israelites, which contained within it both the shards of the Ten Commandments that Moses had broken and the intact tablets that replaced them, the whole of experience and the parts of experience reside in the brains of Alzheimer's patients. The mind is the "Book of Lost Books": knowledge that used to be and ceases to be, a highlighted notation that inexplicably and idiosyncratically repeats, a reference wrongly attributed, a volume in the Book of Life, a particular that gradually becomes generic, a blank slate. Alzheimer's unbinds the diary of our life's experiences and runs it backwards until it runs out, the pages strewn about and the ink of the words on the page faded and illegible. What remains of a word becomes insensible. What remains of our world becomes imperceptible. Our bodies are still intact in the flesh, but our minds are unraveling. What can we make of a phenomenon that causes reality to be illusory and vanishing? Like the Ark with the whole and the parts, the brain can be revealed not only by the orderly chronicling and recall of experience, but by the lapses and disarray that disease renders. One version of the world exists in a continuum, but another has holes. This is the challenge of illness. This is the challenge of Alzheimer's disease.

Alzheimer's Dementia: A History of Terms

Medicine is the art of applying science, control, and order to the inhomogeneous workings of each human being. What we currently understand about dementia, and specifically Alzheimer's disease, derives from a series of verbal and visual portraits, histories of natural observations. As such, medicine exists in the embrace of social forces. The notion of what is disease, and what is not, is colored by societal constructs and myths. Alzheimer's disease and other dementias are most certainly ancient, even though their scientific and eponymous designations may only be a century and a half old. Their first codification may be through folktales, natural history lessons transmitted through the moralistic parables told by grandmothers to very young children.

Isaac Bashevis Singer captures the iconic image of a demented woman in Baba Yaga, the main character of his children's story "Joseph and Koza."[1] The name Baba Yaga evokes the infantilization and diminished function of demented individuals. *Baba* means "old woman" or "grandmother" in most Slavic languages; it echoes the babbling of infants and often carries pejorative connotations in modern use. *Yaga* derives from Proto-Slavic words that mean "lazy," "questioning," or "quarrelsome," completing the personality profile of demented individuals.[2] In the classic folktale, Baba Yaga is pictured as gaunt and disheveled, with the long, curved fingernails of someone who no longer grooms. Her neglected cat, starving dog, and broken gate abandon her as she has abandoned them. Her lost ability to recognize objects leads her to travel by mortar and pestle instead of cart and horse. She speaks to invisible spirits, and when she is questioned by others, it causes her to fly into a rage. She avoids answering questions, it is said, because for every question asked, she ages by one year, a reference to the memory loss associated with advanced age. Her seemingly irrational hunt for plump children to eat while getting lost in a tangled forest is not only a metaphor for trying to find lost youth, but also for the failure of problem solving and executive function. Her solution to the food problem is the same as a modern Alzheimer's patient: a supper of cold, thin soup. Moreover, she lives in the same society we have today, isolated and still stigmatized: "She lived in the woods alone. She ate alone, slept alone, and her loneliness made more bitter by the stories told about her—terrible stories, horrible stories, the terrible horrible Baba Yaga."[3]

The temptation to demonize and isolate those with dementia continued until the very end of the nineteenth century. A German psychiatrist, Dr. Alois Alzheimer, attending to mentally ill patients in Frankfurt's city asylum, observed the curious case of an amnestic fifty-one-year-old woman, Auguste Deter, whose husband deposited her there after she "abandoned" her house, dog, and children. A photo of her reveals a gaunt and disheveled woman. Her nighttime wanderings through the building, screaming and dragging bedsheets, evoked the nocturnal flights of the caped and cackling Baba Yaga. Deluded by failing memory, she chased after others for thefts they didn't commit. Words and objects were insensible; as she ate pork and cauliflower, she remarked that she was chewing spinach. Her answers to Dr. Alzheimer's varied questions were like a babbling incantation: first name, "Auguste"; last name, "Auguste"; husband's name, "Auguste"; and the number eight is written A-U-G-U-S-T-E. Like the wandering Baba Yaga in the forest, she commented, "It seems that I have lost myself."[4] She ate and slept alone, and her loneliness was made bitter as Dr. Alzheimer, unable to control her behaviors, placed her in isolation. Curiously, Dr. Alzheimer recognized these behaviors, for he had observed them in the elderly, but this was the first time he identified them in someone so young.

Mrs. Deter died in April 1906. Not content to merely record another medical curiosity or explain it away, as was the fashion of the time, with the language of Freudian psychology, Dr. Alzheimer investigated the physical basis of Auguste Deter's distinctive cognitive disorder.[5] Utilizing the novel technique of silver staining, he identified the amyloid plaques and neurofibrillary tangles in her brain that have since become the pathological definition of the disease. For the first time, the clinical symptoms of what was termed "presenile dementia" were grounded in pathological alterations of the brain.

Despite Alois Alzheimer's scientific recasting of Baba Yaga in 1906 as the neurological disorder that today carries his name, the term "Alzheimer's dementia" remained a separate and shunned category of cognitive impairment. The birth of the disorder in an insane asylum by a specialist in mental disorders did not enhance its credibility. Clinicians may have avoided the label and dismissed the parallels between "presenile" and "senile" dementia at least in part due to fear—the terrible, horrible connotation of Alzheimer's disease. Like cancer, another disease whose origins couldn't be understood, the term "Alzheimer's" was to be uttered, if at all, only in whispers. The lack of coherence between the Alzheimer's of the young and the dementia of the aged colored the scientific and medical approaches to diagnosis and classification of dementing disorders. Physicians distinguished "presenile" from "senile dementia": the former describing dementia occurring before age sixty-five and related to Alzheimer's pathology, but the latter casting almost a pejorative label for cognitive decline related to the aging process alone. In the mid-1980s, scientists rediscovered the plaques and tangles of Alzheimer's dementia, but this time they identified them in the brains of aged individuals. Clinicians then merged the two separate categories, presenile and senile Alzheimer's dementia, into the designation "senile dementia of the Alzheimer's type." This singular designation underwent another split in the 1990s, as geneticists identified autosomal dominant mutations in genes associated with individuals who develop Alzheimer's disease before age sixty, but a different set of genes and risk factors in those with Alzheimer's disease after age sixty. This time clinicians abandoned the pejoratives and coined the terms "early onset" for Alzheimer's disease before age sixty and "late onset" for that after age sixty.

Alzheimer's disease and many other primary degenerative dementias increase in frequency with age. Although willing to concede that some elderly individuals developed Alzheimer's disease, clinicians still allowed for a category of individuals with diminished capacity who, they believed, suffered simply from a normal surcease of brain function.

Many schemas were developed to try to distinguish normal memory loss of aging from dementia: if you lost something and knew it was lost, it wasn't dementia; however, if you lost something and didn't know that it was lost, it was dementia. This worked only if you applied the criteria once; over time, persons who fell in the first category had a tendency to thereafter fall into the latter category. Also, by the time someone did not know that they did not know, all insight was lost, and those individuals would not seek medical attention. Other problems arose from the theory that aging alone caused mental demise. Like Jean Clemente, who lived for 122 years and 134 days without dementia, how could one explain the 30 to 40 percent of people living beyond 100 years who never develop cognitive decline, despite their advanced age?

The idea of normal surcease in cognitive function was challenged by clinical-pathological studies that identified abnormal brain pathologies occurring to some degree in individuals who possessed cognitive change of any degree. Conforming to the research, physicians gradually adopted the notion that changes in thinking were abnormal, not an accompaniment of normal aging, and more commonly applied the term "dementia" to individuals with thinking problems. Dementia itself, though, was defined based on the characteristics of the most common dementing disorder of the elderly, Alzheimer's disease. "Dementia" is an umbrella term for any disorder of cognition. Until recently, however, the term "dementia" was conflated with Alzheimer's. Since Alzheimer's presents with memory loss as the most salient symptom, the umbrella term "dementia" required memory loss. The other causes of dementia, for example, Lewy body dementia or frontotemporal dementia, do not affect memory early or in the same way as Alzheimer's disease. Therefore, many dementias went undiagnosed or were diagnosed in very advanced stages. Although none of the major neurodegenerative dementias can be cured, medical treatments and the course of disease differ among them, and for this reason alone, it is important to distinguish between them. In addition, in order for curative treatments to be developed, clinical diagnostic criteria need to be defined to accurately differentiate the dementias so experimental treatments may target the appropriate group.

New diagnostic criteria created in 2010 redefine dementia to designate significant impairment in any two domains of cognitive function, therefore not necessarily requiring memory loss. It is also possible for Alzheimer's disease to present without significant memory loss, at least until much later. Particularly in individuals whose disease begins in their thirties to sixties, language impairment, visual processing impairment, or impairment in executive function, a group of functions related to the selection and deployment of a number of brain processes needed for problem solving, may predominate. Clinical criteria for the dementias in essence create portraits, descriptive behavioral characteristics for each disorder. The assumption is that there is a single underlying pathology related to each set of characteristics. What we now know is that any dementia is a clinical syndrome; that is, its clinical characteristics result from a combination of pathological insults to the brain. How each pathological change leads to clinical manifestations and why and in what way pathologies interact still need to be determined.

Clinicians may apply the common, undifferentiated term "dementia" to denote the milder symptoms of early stages of Alzheimer's disease, and then only when symptoms worsen might they label the disorder as Alzheimer's. Presently, we know that one does not just wake up one day with Alzheimer's disease. A cascade of alterations in brain structures and function evolves over decades. New imaging technologies of whole brain structure and function, and the application of mathematical models to brain function, elucidate the slow changes that underlie an asymptomatic preclinical stage, as well as early declines in several domains of thinking called mild cognitive impairment, and finally the rapidly progressive and unrelenting dementia stages that are divided into mild, moderate, and severe. All stages are in effect Alzheimer's *disease*, that is, they are all due to a group of pathologies that specifically target one network in the brain that gives rise to the specific symptoms of Alzheimer's disease. Dementia is the end result of a series of stresses that ultimately overwhelm the brain's ability to compensate and leads to a progressive downward spiral. The diagnostic criteria for dementia and

Alzheimer's disease released in 2010 reflect this new understanding of dementia and Alzheimer's disease.

The current concept of the evolution of Alzheimer's dementia includes a long prodrome of changes in the brain before any symptoms appear, called preclinical disease. Biomarkers, fingerprints of dementia such as changes in cerebrospinal fluid proteins, volume changes, and loss of connections in and between critical areas of brain function, now exist to identify these different stages. By identifying pathological changes earlier and knowing more about their causes and how they disrupt normal brain networks and overcome compensatory mechanisms, researchers may be able to devise preventive or disease-modifying treatments. Curiously, these technologies reveal that some individuals harbor severe levels of Alzheimer's or other dementia pathologies, yet never develop cognitive decline. This suggests that there are genetic or environmental factors that counteract the negative effects of brain pathologies, which, if identified, could be applied to help people function even if Alzheimer's disease cannot be prevented or cured.

Perhaps the old stories of infantilized witches, Baba Yaga, can be put to bed. Cognitive history can now be revised. Old age is not senility. Pathology is not destiny. We may find our way out of the tangled woods.

The Tangled Woods

Storytelling reflects biological functions, and it must serve an adaptive function. The metaphors of stories may also arise from universal biological structures. It is probably no accident, for instance, that Creation stories across cultures illustrate knowledge in the form of a tree. Woods, trees, branches, leaves, and roots not only stand on their own as biological systems, but they also serve as representations of the structure of human thought. The human inventions of paper and books also serve as extended tree metaphors for living systems, perhaps the most notable being the Book of Life. The word "book," a depository for knowledge and memory, derives from the Indo-European root word for birch tree. Birch bark served as one of the earliest materials for paper. Creation myths utilize trees to symbolize knowledge.

Isaac Bashevis Singer writes that "if stories weren't told or books weren't written, man would live like the beasts, only for a day."[6] A story is a store for memory, a tool to contain and disseminate knowledge even before books existed, an oral law even before a written law. One distinction of humankind from animals is the story, collective memory, a survival tool that surpasses the inborn instincts of all other beings. That the human brain seems to relish the structure and patterns of stories suggests that it is inherent in the design of our brain to discern and configure narratives and search them for meaning. Then, once aware of an overarching theme, it constructs a moral, a rule that guides behavior. Judaism depends on those mental stratagems of story making and rule formation; it relates knowledge via midrashim and impels action by mitzvot. Stories make us aware so we may act—from midrash to mitzvah.

Stories cannot exist without memory. Memory allows a reference to past experience that serves as a guide to the present and future. We don't just take in information; we screen it, sift it, sort it, strip it down to its bare bones, and then recast it on the larger armature of the rest of what we know. It has meaning only when it relates to the rest of what we know. Memory therefore begins as a sensory trace, an awareness of something experienced in the world outside of us by means of our four senses. Sensory information is not just registered into our conscious brains, but is analyzed, broken down into component parts, related to other current and past sensory traces, reconfigured, and then funneled to a common repository, called memory, located in the hippocampus in the temporal lobe of the brain. Here, the experience is recorded in permanent ink, long-term memory, a page in our book of life, a journal, a catalogue of our personal experiences, the what, the where, and the order of when it all happened. It is a highly idiosyncratic log of life, but it serves as a reference to whatever else we may encounter. It is our own story and told from our own perspective. We revisit it, and throughout our whole lives, we revise it. It records all the time that we are awake but then needs sleep to withdraw the antennas on the outside world so it can retreat to the archives of our past experiences and derive meaning from the mass of incoming data. Experiences are not only literally solidified in new connections between appropriate nerve cells during successive stages of sleep, but they become enmeshed in the fabric of previous experience. In other words, links are made from new bits of information to old bits of information based on shared sensory characteristics of those experiences. Meaning derives from the intermingling of past with present. And to manage the morass of information, the brain creates collections of data, categories, to organize seemingly random facts and experience into understandable, sensible groups. That which something is, relates to what it is like. In our minds, then, life is a continuous simile and all the similes, our stories.

But we do die. We often decay and decline before we die. We are a tree planted outside the garden. This is God's prophecy of Alzheimer's disease.

In the Baba Yaga story, there is a moment when youth encounters old age; the young girl throws down a comb and from it grows a forest. But it is already a tangled forest, a forest in winter. While hopefully and hungrily chasing the child, Baba Yaga encounters obstacles, metaphorical tangles in thinking just like the tangles of Alzheimer's disease. So consumed by the effort of the pursuit, she loses the reason for the pursuit, metaphorically losing the forest for the trees. Alzheimer's is like a tree in winter. It is the end point—often just when a diagnosis is first being made, a tree stripped bare of leaves and branches, no longer capable of making new connections, bereft of old connections, and in a downward self-perpetuating spiral of neuronal death. There is bark still on the tree, but there is neither scribe nor ink to mark time and experience on its surface.

In the spring, the brain expands its networks and connections, it leafs out the branches and then grows a robust summer growth of new associations and connections. Imperceptibly at first, autumn appears. The tree starts to die. New leaves fail to keep up with the loss of leaves. Ramifications diminish. Perhaps someone complains that their memory is failing, or maybe there is slight unease and anxiety without any specific awareness of memory loss. Perhaps no symptom is yet present. This is the beginning of the fall.

This is the season to tend to our tree and our garden.

PART II

Adaptation

8

⁂

Doorways of Hope: Adapting to Alzheimer's

SHELDON MARDER

"Be assured," says God,
"I will . . . lead [Israel] through the wilderness
and I will speak to her with tenderness.
I will give her vineyards . . .
and [I will give her] the Valley of Achor
as a doorway of hope. . . ."

—Hosea 2:16–17[1]

In the eighth century BCE, the Valley of Achor was an arid waste-land—"a valley of trouble"—and for the prophet Hosea it served as an apt symbol of Israel's spiritual condition at the time. In a place of despair, says the prophet, God will bring forth vineyards as a sign of the land's vitality, goodness, and abundance, and Achor will become a *petach tikvah*—a doorway of hope.

I believe, as did Hosea, that hope can take root in any soil. I believe that we have the capacity to experience God's presence in places of suffering and unease.

Robert Davis, minister of a large church in Miami, describes his experience of one such "place" in a book called *My Journey into Alzheimer's Disease*. What does Alzheimer's feel like? Davis writes:

> [There is] the devastation of losing self-confidence, parts of the old independent personality, memory, pride as I became a care receiver instead of a care giver. . . . The worst personal loss was the

77

spiritual change that suddenly came to me. . . . At night when it is total blackness, these absurd fears come. The comforting memories can't be reached. The mind-sustaining Bible verses are gone. The old emotions are gone as new, uncontrolled, fearful emotions sweep in to replace them. The sweetness of prayer and the gentle comfort of [God] are gone. I am alone in the blackness. . . . I personally discovered the full meaning of what the psalmist called "the terror by night" (Ps. 91:5).[2]

A woman in her midforties told this story about her descent into dementia: "One day, while out for a walk on my usual path in a city in which I had resided for 11 years, nothing looked familiar. It was as if I was lost in a foreign land."[3]

These are frightening accounts; but the purpose of this chapter is not to instill fear—rather, the opposite. The proposition I want to explore is this: there are doorways of hope in the alien, terrifying land of dementia. In the face of catastrophic illness, Jewish tradition can provide sustenance: vitality, goodness, and strength. No, these doors are not easily opened. And, yes, concepts like vitality and goodness take on relative meaning. Nevertheless, I believe there are ways to find comfort, meaning, and moments of spiritual healing for ourselves and the people we care for. Alzheimer's, by definition, will distance us from our normal lives, but it need not distance us from God's presence.

Let me give you an example. A man named Jonah[4] moved into the Jewish Home a few years ago, and I immediately felt an affinity for him. Like many of our residents, Jonah had multiple chronic illnesses; the most serious was Parkinson's disease, which was accompanied by a profound, disorienting dementia. When I first met him, however, Jonah was able to tell me about himself and his most important interests: his family, his religious life in Chicago, and his productive years in Israel. Having attended every Shabbat service for a year, Jonah failed to appear one Saturday morning. When I asked a nurse why Jonah had not been brought to services, she replied, "He's gotten so disoriented, he doesn't know where he is. He doesn't even know that he lives here in G-3." I said, "You're right. He has no idea what G-3 is. But when he's in the synagogue, he knows *exactly* where he is." What

Jonah needed was a tallis around his shoulders and the soft chant of psalms and blessings. In the warm intimacy of communal worship, Jonah was in his element; he was in God's presence—and he knew it.

But most of the time it is not that simple. We need to acknowledge that all talk about faith, hope, and God is problematic when dementia enters the picture. Alzheimer's disease is relentless in putting our religion and our theologies to the test. One writer has even named Alzheimer's the "theological disease" because of the fierce challenges it poses to our beliefs about what it means to be a human being created by God.[5]

For Jews in particular, dementia raises thorny theological issues. Especially troublesome is our self-image as "the people of the Book"— a people for whom learning and literacy are central. What happens to a Jew who can no longer read the book? What becomes of her relationship to the Jewish people, to Jewish history, and to God when the Bible and the Haggadah are out of reach?

In the Jewish Home's synagogue, people with dementia hold the prayer book, though they cannot decipher it. They clutch it close, turn and crumple its pages; they drop it to the floor and reach for it. I am moved as I observe the physical expressions of their attachment to the prayer book, and I am saddened that the priority we give to the written word pushes them to the margins of our religion.

Thorny issue #2: According to Maimonides, when God said, "Let us make Adam in our image," God was referring to the intellect.[6] Our likeness to God, he said, is not physical; it is mental. Does this mean that the person with dementia becomes, in the course of his illness, an increasingly flawed and "fading image of God"?[7] Is he still an image of God at all—a reflection of holiness and divinity? Or does cognitive failure—the failure to apprehend the world intellectually—mean that this person is no longer *b'tzelem Elohim*, a creature made in God's image?

The third issue is the loss of memory. What is the Jewish religion without the memory of the Exodus from Egypt? Appearing 169 times in the Bible, the verb *zachar* (remember) is a constant reminder that the covenant between Israel and God depends on the act of remembering. What is Judaism without *Yizkor* and *Kaddish*? Who are we if we no longer remember the Sabbath day to keep it holy? The mitzvah to empathize with the stranger, widow, and orphan is based on our ability to remember our people's experience as strangers.

What is a Jew—what is a human being—when loss of memory deprives a person of these values and wellsprings of connection? As one writer has put it, "With the loss of memory goes the loss of faith."[8] Can Jewish faith survive when memory is damaged or lost entirely? And how do other Jews regard the spirituality of a person with memory loss?

We are a people of the book, a people of intellect, a people of memory. Learning and remembrance have been our survival strategies for centuries. But we also have to recognize that these strategies—which place the mind at the center of religious life—cannot function for a Jew facing dementia.

What else does our tradition have to offer?

In a small gem of a book about Jewish spirituality, Rabbi Samuel Dresner takes the emphasis off the mind and directs our attention to another precious sign of the image of God: the human soul. He writes:

> Man is like a cord tied at two ends: bound to the earth through his body and to heaven through his soul. He is partly animal through the physical aspect of his being and partly angel through the spiritual aspect of his being. He is mortal yet immortal, transient yet eternal, filled at once with misery and grandeur.[9]

Rabbi Dresner wrote those words in 1957, when Alzheimer's disease was relatively unknown, even to doctors. Medical school textbooks of that era called it "pre-senile dementia." Though not writing with this disease in mind, Rabbi Dresner speaks to the heart of my everyday experience of people with dementia. They are bound to the earth by their bodies and to heaven by their souls; part animal, part angel, they are filled with misery and with grandeur.

How, then, do we touch the soul, the divine element in every human being? How can we find the grandeur amidst so much misery? I have discovered no better way to do this than through poetry. A poem can change the way we see our world; and, in the valley of despair, even subtle shifts in perception can transform one's perspective. In addition, a poem's metaphors invite intimacy.[10]

For example, Psalm 23 encourages us to reframe our emotional landscape; it offers a vision of goodness, vitality, and abundance when we feel overwhelmed by enemies, darkness, and fear. Through the psalm's images and reframing, we discover refreshment for the soul and the ability to say to God, "Thou art with me" even here, even in this place.

Some poems touch the soul of the person who is ill; others speak powerfully to family and caregivers. A poem like David Mason's "The Inland Sea" can even dare to suggest that there is beauty and dignity in Alzheimer's:

> Their dignity another universe
> might honor more than we do, seeing souls
> where we see bodies failing into death. . . .
> Their beauty terrifies us, so we think
> it like no beauty we have ever known
> and leave them for the ordinary shore.[11]

Some poems transport us mysteriously to places of beauty. Others, like Psalm 23, transform the way we see ourselves and our situation. In diverse ways, poetry can be a doorway of hope in the valley of trouble. With that in mind, we turn to a poem by poet laureate Billy Collins:

Forgetfulness

> The name of the author is the first to go
> followed obediently by the title, the plot,
> the heartbreaking conclusion, the entire novel
> which suddenly becomes one you have never read,
> never even heard of,

as if, one by one, the memories you used to harbor
decided to retire to the southern hemisphere of the brain,
to a little fishing village where there are no phones.

Long ago you kissed the names of the nine Muses goodbye
and watched the quadratic equation pack its bag,
and even now as you memorize the order of the planets,
something else is slipping away, a state flower perhaps,
the address of an uncle, the capital of Paraguay.

Whatever it is you are struggling to remember
it is not poised on the tip of your tongue,
not even lurking in some obscure corner of your spleen.

It has floated away down a dark mythological river
whose name begins with an *L* as far as you can recall,
well on your way to oblivion where you will join those
who have even forgotten how to swim and how to ride a bicycle.

No wonder you rise in the middle of the night
to look up the date of a famous battle in a book on war.
No wonder the moon in the window seems to have drifted
out of a love poem that you used to know by heart.[12]

With some trepidation, I read "Forgetfulness" with a group of twenty elders—residents of the Jewish Home, ages eighty to one hundred. Two or three members of the group had Alzheimer's disease; two were married to people with Alzheimer's.

I read the poem aloud. When I finished, there was silence, and I could feel some discomfort in the room. So I asked a playful question to get the ball rolling: "Who knows the capital of Paraguay?" As it happened, only one person knew the answer. Morrie, a former social studies teacher who has Alzheimer's disease, replied, "Asunción." His tone was impatient, as if I were wasting his time with such an easy question. Morrie not only got the right answer; he drew a gasp of amazement from the group—and even a laugh, which broke the ice.

Morrie's response opened a floodgate of feelings from others in the group. The elders talked about the meaning of forgetfulness in their lives as they age: the embarrassment, the problems it causes, their feelings of self-doubt. Most important, they spoke in confessional tones about fear of diseases that cause the dementia they see around them in the nursing home. With its gentle wit, a poem like "Forgetfulness" helps us face our fears and, perhaps, embrace a part of ourselves we tend to deny.[13]

Judy, a person at an early stage of Alzheimer's, did not speak during the class but afterwards approached me with urgency and excitement. "Rabbi," she said, "that's me. That's exactly how *I* feel. It's like the phones are cut off. I'm always forgetting everything. Thank you. Thank you. It was so good to hear everyone talk about their feelings."

Judy's touching response to the poem and the discussion teaches us several important lessons.

First: We touch the soul of the person with dementia through acts of empathy and compassion. We learn from Judy that the sharing of feelings (rather than silence, a more typical response to Alzheimer's) can bring comfort and sustenance to a person in distress. It is the sure feeling that other people understand what we are going through. And that's what Judy felt.

The psychiatrist Milton H. Erickson gave a name to the kind of sharing the poem encouraged. Erickson called it "joining the patient."[14] Joining the patient means entering his world, trying to feel what he feels, expressing yourself in his language, joining in the playfulness. As one daughter of a mother with Alzheimer's writes, "In Mother's company, I had to be more alive than I had ever been. . . . We were often silly together, as when her Boston terrier, Anne, jumped into the bath with her, and we decided to just go ahead and bathe her too, Mother calling for me to get the camera because she didn't want to forget it."[15]

In our discussion of the poem, Judy heard other people describe their forgetfulness as a frightening, embarrassing part of their lives. Without realizing it, they were joining themselves to Judy, speaking to her soul, attaching their concerns to hers. Through their empathy, Judy felt keenly that they were "on her side," as she later told me.

The technique of "joining the patient" is even more effective when it is used intentionally, and that intention is clear throughout the Torah, where we find that "joining the stranger"—understanding those who are vulnerable—is a sacred obligation. As stated in Exodus 23:9, "You shall not oppress a stranger, for you know the soul [the feelings] of the stranger, having been strangers yourselves in the land of Egypt."

We touch the soul of a person with dementia through acts of empathy and compassion.

Second: We touch the soul through the work of sustaining relationships. Depending on the stage of the illness, it can be hard just to have a conversation. A person with dementia speaks in non sequiturs, cannot think of words, rarely asks you personal questions, and sometimes doesn't speak at all. There is no easy and natural interchange; the awkward silence is overwhelming.

The fundamental material for conversation is often lacking, because a person with dementia cannot make new memories. He is unable to tell you what he ate for lunch; she does not remember your visit that morning. Without a sense of continuity and shared memories, just finding something to say can be an exhausting challenge.

Most important, in the presence of a loved one who has Alzheimer's, we often find ourselves overwhelmed by our own emotions: disappointment, sadness, frustration, anger, fear. We keep imagining how horrible this must be for them, because we cannot help thinking how humiliating it would be for us—to have to be fed, to have to wear diapers. The prospect is terrifying for us. A woman told me about seeing her mother dancing with a staff member at her nursing home. "Imagine!" she said. "*My* mother—who was always so dignified, private, and reserved—my mother, making a fool of herself on the dance floor. How could they do that to her?"

Thoughts like these can be so painful that we find it excruciating to be with a loved one who has dementia; we're counting the minutes until we can leave. Sustaining relationships under these conditions takes patience, persistence, and imagination. But I know it is possible, and I know it can make a significant difference. Here are a few guidelines.

Joining the patient means entering into his world without inhibition and recognizing that he is now a different person. A fastidious, reserved woman may now enjoy dancing in a funny hat; a loving husband can become disagreeable, uttering curse words you never heard come out of his mouth. We only torment ourselves if we keep comparing our loved one with the way he or she used to be. We have to face the fact that we are now forming a relationship with a new person—indeed, a person who continues to change over time, as the illness develops.

Realize that the person with dementia does not feel the way you think you would if you were in that situation. He does not find the silence awkward. She is not suffering from indignities that would cause you pain. In order to be with your loved one, you have to let go of your feelings and accept who this person is. When you can let go of your feelings, you can have happy moments—peaceful, enjoyable moments with your loved one—and there is healing for both of you.

We learn from Judy's experience that dementia can feel like "the phones are cut off." In other words, lines of communication are frayed and disappearing; isolation is an ever-present danger. Still, Judy continued to attend classes and services, danced whenever she heard music, and enjoyed the songwriting workshop. "It was good to hear everyone," she said.

Judy's yearning for relationship reminds us of God's words in Genesis 2:18, regarding Adam's situation as a solitary human being: "It is not good for a person to be alone." So God created Eve. Our tradition understands that relationship with other people is at the heart of our existence. Loss of brain cells does not alter this fundamental human need.

We touch the soul through acts of empathy and compassion and through sustaining relationships.

Third: I learned from Judy that a poem—an expression of imagination and creativity—is a powerful way to open the door to a person with dementia. One reason for this is that people with dementia often speak in metaphor. Like poets, they use unusual words and images to mean something else; for example, the man who looked down at his own feet and told his son, "They're gonna be trees."[16]

In fact, the language of dementia shares quite a few qualities with poetry: its ambiguity; the way it leaps and flows in a nonlinear, associative way; and especially the fact that the metaphoric language requires thoughtful interpretation on our part. What did that man mean when he said his feet are "gonna be trees"? The skill of interpretation that we develop by reading poetry can help us understand people with dementia. And what's more, poetry sensitizes us to the human condition. This is why one poet says that "the best poetry depends on an intensity of empathy. . . . The poetry I love most . . . makes me feel the condition of another."[17]

People with dementia have the ability to respond to creative writing. In fact, the poem can awaken their creativity. Almost any image will elicit a response that gives us a glimpse into a person's soul and inner feelings.

This happened in an impromptu discussion in which I used a poem called "Tiny Joys" by the Hebrew poet Rachel.[18] The poem begins, "Tiny joys, joys like a lizard's tail . . ." I asked the group why they think the poet repeats the word "joys." Someone said, "To remember it." Another person gave the phrase "tiny joys" a whole new feeling when she said, "I prefer to think of them as 'little pleasures.'" And someone else made the observation that "*all* joys are big—no joy is tiny." To which another participant added, "The *tail* is tiny . . . the joy is important . . . the joy is *big*." I decided to use my knowledge of Jonah (mentioned above), asking him, "Jonah, didn't taking photographs give you joy?" And Jonah responded, "Yes, it did give me a certain amount of joy to take photographs of the land." And I followed up, "Jonah, when you say 'land,' you mean Israel, right?" "Yes, Israel," Jonah said. "Israel gives me joy." The poem helps us touch the deepest part of a person.

Creativity is the third doorway of hope—the third way to touch the soul. Of course it also happens through music and art, and it is a very Jewish way. Think for a moment about the opening verses of Genesis.

I remember once reflecting on various ways that the Bible could begin: with a prayer, perhaps; with a statement of faith, like the 23rd Psalm; or with the great moment at Mount Sinai—to name just a few possibilities. But none of these was chosen as chapter one. *B'reishit bara Elohim*, "When God began to create . . ." God's first act in the Bible is Creation. Bezalel, the creator of the Tabernacle, is filled with "the spirit of God" (Exodus 31:3). A Jewish Home resident said to me, "The art room is my reason for staying alive." We learn from our texts and we learn from our experience that embedded within Judaism is this profound truth: creativity is primary; creativity is the essence of life.

Hannah, ninety years old, with dementia, was actively dying. There were long periods of sleep, and there were times when she would wake up agitated and confused. Although Hannah was a lifelong, native English speaker, she was now speaking only in short Yiddish phrases during these episodes of discomfort, and it was clear to her daughter that Hannah was speaking in Yiddish to one person: her grandmother. For Hannah, Yiddish was the *mama loshen* (mother tongue); her first memories of her grandmother were in Yiddish.

We know that people with dementia often return to a language learned early in life. And yet, I could not help but wonder if there was something more specific happening deep inside Hannah. The more I listened to her, the more I thought there might be. As I told her daughter, I could feel Hannah's soul turning to the most reliable source of comfort she had ever known in her life: the grandmother who raised her as a child. Now, in her last days, Hannah's soul "remembered" exactly what she needed. She remembered the right words, the right language, and the right person. Hannah had become her own spiritual healer. When I said this to Hannah's daughter, she cried and told me that this brought her comfort.

If we gaze long and carefully at a person with dementia, sometimes we are able to see that person in a new way, to reframe and reinterpret what is happening inside that person, just as we Jews are taught to do with a sacred text. Hannah was my sacred text. I was honored to help her daughter read that text in a creative, empathic way that connected her to the generations of her family.

Those are my three doorways into the land of dementia, my three suggestions for touching the divine soul of the man or woman in the valley of trouble: empathy, relationship, creativity. Each doorway is a *petach tikvah*—an opening of hope. None of these doorways depends on the learning, literacy, and memory so central to the Judaism most of us practice. Therefore, I want to suggest that dementia requires a different kind of Judaism.

Poet Tess Gallagher, who was the caregiver throughout her mother's seventeen years of Alzheimer's, writes that she and her mother achieved something surprising during that time: "We moved beyond forgetting. . . . From stage to stage I kept insisting, until I did manage to stimulate both doctors and caregivers toward the sense that, even though her condition might be 'hopeless' in the ultimate sense of what medicine could offer, there were still unexplored things we could do to make life better for her."[19]

Tess hoped for something better for her mother: a life that was less confusing, more secure, and more attentive to her mother's feelings. Their relationship illustrates what the literature on dementia calls "habilitative care."[20] The goal of rehabilitation is to restore abilities and skills in a person who has lost them. Habilitative care is life-affirming and hopeful, focusing on preserving what remains: a person who can paint or knit or enjoy word games is encouraged to do these activities regularly; missing one day of activity can mean losing the skill forever. Hebrew has a title for people like Tess, spiritual caregivers who tend to the souls of others. We call them *k'lei kodesh*—"vessels of holiness"—people for whom caregiving is more "calling" than obligation.

Empathy, relationship, and creativity: these are the ingredients of a Judaism that is habilitative for people with dementia—a Judaism that can help sustain a person's connection to self and others, as long as possible. Rather than allow Judaism to fail us when we need it most, habilitative Judaism—with a focus on touching the soul—makes our religion relevant in our care for people with dementia.

After twenty years of illness, my father's final diagnosis was dementia with Lewy bodies. He spent his last few years at the Jewish Home, happily creating colorful abstract paintings in the art room. My father had two passions beyond his work as a lawyer; art was one of them, and reading was the other.

Sometime in the middle of his illness, he asked a favor of me, something my father rarely did: he wanted me to drive him to the public library. A voracious reader all his life, my father had taken me to the library almost every weekend for years when I was a child. On each visit, he would sign out a tall stack of books; he read them all.

The library had been my father's sanctuary, his holy of holies. Now, in the middle of his dementia—after a break of thirty-five years—we were making a weekly pilgrimage to the library.

This library was small, a safe place for a person with dementia to wander around; lots of people wander in the stacks. I stationed myself near the door, so he could not get lost. As in the old days, he would sign out a tall stack of books. But now he was unable to read them.

One morning, during one of these outings, my father became very serious and said he wanted to tell me something about his illness. I remember it clearly; it happened only once. And this is what he said: "Shelly, I feel as though there is a veil between me and the rest of the world. Everything seems hazy. I just can't break through the veil."

My father couldn't break through the veil—his illness wouldn't let him. I cried when he said those words to me. I cried because I realized how upset he was, and because my father hardly ever shared his deepest feelings with me. I realized that he was giving me the best gift, the only gift he could offer me in the midst of his anguish and fear. My father was opening his heart. He could not break through, but he was inviting me to join him behind the veil.

Ever since that day, I have been trying to figure out how to do that, searching for ways we can join the people we love in their loneliness and solitude behind the veil. After many years of trying, I know it is possible. Given enough time and patience and compassion, we can find a way in. We can remain in relationship, even as life changes and illness progresses. We can continue to see the image of God within the human being before us. Even in dark places, there can be moments of beauty and dignity. Believe me when I tell you: there are openings in the veil—doorways of hope.

9

🍃

Let There Be Light:
Creative Adaptations to Alzheimer's

MINA FRIEDLER

And God said, "Let there be light!—and there was light."
—Genesis 1:3

The essential key to unlocking the world in which people with Alzheimer's disease and other dementias are living is to step into their universe and try to experience it through their eyes, without fear, condescension, or judgment. In this way, their perceptions mingle with ours and become tools for unlocking our own potential to understand the vast spectrum of humanity. In this way, we keep the flame of their cognition and memory burning as long as we can.

In order to create light where light seems to be dimming, we must first realize that, as Genesis teaches, we are all made in the image of God (Genesis 1:26). According to the late Lubavitcher Rebbe Menachem Mendel Schneerson, the four species that are shaken in the *lulav* on Sukkot represent the entire Jewish people, for without each and every one—including those with physical and mental perspectives different than our own—the unity of *K'lal Yisrael*, all of Israel, would not be possible.

How do we adapt to a capricious reality that seems to be robbing our loved ones of what is most precious, namely, memory? My experience suggests it is by seeking out the unique desires, yearnings, and potential for and expressions of actualization—for fulfillment of oneself—that exist in all of us. By using art, music, movement, and poetry, revisiting the familiar in unfamiliar ways, exchanging knowledge between generations, and mentoring those less fortunate than ourselves, we can illuminate the darkness and seek that fulfillment of actualization, even in those with dementia.

To Draw Out One's Voice

Memory is a collection of experiences, perceptions, pictures, yearnings, and desires. However, many of these yearnings and desires remain unrealized during life because their actualization threatens our self-perceptions within the social context we occupy, and life's hectic demands and responsibilities do not allow for such fulfillment to occur. Both metaphorically and emotionally, Alzheimer's disease causes time to freeze at the very same moment that the diseased person's inhibitions are eroding. This dialectic of unrealized desires and eroding inhibitions creates an optimum condition for new forms of artistic expression to emerge. In the middle stage of Alzheimer's disease, when cognition is still at a relatively high level, a person is often able to express frustrations and fears through the creative process. Alzheimer's makes the present moment more real, because the past, due to fading memory, is diminished. Inhibitions begin to erode, and desires and yearning are left raw and open.

I met Jackie, an accomplished clinical psychologist, on the first day I began work as an activity coordinator for a senior program for frail elderly at the Jewish Community Center in Los Angeles. She sat, tall and regal, at a long table covered with stencils of flowers, crayons strewn about. Women and men in their seventies and eighties were busily coloring in the lines, blank looks on their faces. I smiled at Jackie. She scowled back at me. "I hate this," she said, pointing at the stencils and the crayons. "Just because I have Alzheimer's doesn't mean I'm a child. I'm an adult." She told me she had no desire for busy work, to fill in the blanks. She scowled into my eyes, defiant, frustrated, almost in tears.

"What do you want to do?" I asked.

"I want to be free to express myself in my own way," Jackie responded.

The next time we did our art, I told everyone, "This is your opportunity to be whoever you want to be. The paper is your floor. Dance across the years of your life, as you want. You have the freedom to draw your voice." I brought white paper, handmade paper, glue, and paints and oil pastels in a variety of colors—lots of colors. I put the pile of materials in the middle of the table, played Vivaldi's *Four Seasons*, and waited.

"What do you want us to do?" Jackie and some of the other members asked.

"What do you want to do?" I asked in reply.

In the Talmudic tradition, it is customary to answer a question with another question. It is the way we learn. However, via formal cognition is not the only way we learn, and moreover, and perhaps radically, even people with Alzheimer's disease can still ask questions, can still learn, and can still develop new skills. Sometimes, people ask questions without verbally or intellectually asking. Just as a blind or deaf person develops other senses in order to compensate for sensory loss, similarly a person with Alzheimer's often will develop new tools for managing or expressing. Because long-term memory may remain intact up until the end stage of Alzheimer's, these new tools arise out of earlier experiences. For example, a person with dementia who wishes to create a visual, artistic image, drawing on earlier experiences with color and motion, may experiment with different colors as well as movements. A person who has always wanted to drum, recalling a distant concert where a particular drumming sound impressed him, may attempt to replicate that earlier, memorable experience through the mechanism of his own voice.

For the first few minutes, nobody in the room moved. I had experienced this same reticent reaction with other groups of people with cognitive deficiencies, so I was prepared. People who have become accustomed to passively responding to directions often take a while to regain their initiative.

I left the room to do other tasks. When I returned, Jackie had chosen a red marker and was filling her paper with quick, intense strokes.

As Vivaldi's *Four Seasons* gained momentum, so did Jackie's fingers. After filling four sheets of paper, Jackie stopped, her forehead shining with sweat and her face with joy. I looked over her shoulder: in long, graceful strokes, as if her fingers were dancing, she had drawn a series of pictures of three figures holding hands and dancing—a house, a flower, and a garden. I could feel the pulse of her life, her voice, her individuality expressed in color, motion, and music.

Over the next few weeks, I put her pictures together and I realized that they told the story of a mother, father, and child living their lives, happy, contented, and sometimes sad. Other members of the group drew strange figures: babies with wizened, old faces in baby carriages, railroad tracks, automobiles without wheels. They were drawing their lives: individual lives, flames lit separately, a part of yet apart from, putting the pieces of their lives together, compensating for eroding memory through the images on the paper.

As facilitator of the Senior Chai Program for frail elderly at the Westside Jewish Community Center in Los Angeles, my job is to help the people who put themselves in my care to live lives of purpose, joy, and hope for as long as they can. We sometimes arrive to our life callings in strange, yet wondrous ways. Although I had trained to become a labor lawyer, a single event changed my life.

More than twenty years ago, my husband, a geriatric psychiatrist, and I spent our first Rosh HaShanah after we were married worshiping at the Chabad House in Santa Monica, California. At the end of the service, the late Rabbi Levitansky, who conducted the service, asked, "Who can blow the shofar? We need people to blow the shofar for the sick and elderly in convalescent hospitals nearby." My new husband, Eli, whose father had been *rosh yeshivah* (head of the school) of Yeshiva Samson Raphael Hirsch/Broyers, the German-Jewish yeshivah in the Washington Heights neighborhood in New York, had learned to blow the shofar at a very young age. This was customary for young Jewish men in his community. Eli was quick to raise his hand.

Soon, a long train of holiday-garbed young women, children, elderly ladies, men with *shofarot*, rabbis in long black coats with big smiles, and an assortment of street people headed down the street to a nearby convalescent center. Cheerful and heady with the joy of Rosh HaShanah and the California sunshine, we walked down stark, fluorescent-lit corridors, into disinfectant-scented rooms, and we blew the shofar. Each *t'kiah* brought smiles and tears. Old people with dim eyes came alive.

That day, I touched work-worn hands and cheeks where every wrinkle was a museum masterpiece, telling a life story. I whispered, "I love you," to people with Alzheimer's who inhabited a shroud of silence. Yet, it was the shofar, the familiar sound to hungry ears, that opened doors to so many hearts that festival day.

"I remember my mother . . . my father . . . eating at the table . . . I want to blow as I once blew, to hear, to follow . . ."

Personally, I felt that I had come home, that I wanted only to reach inside these people and find a way to help make their lives meaningful once again. Labor law would be someone else's calling; I had found my own. Now, every morning, I hear the shofar in my memory, and I am awakened.

Poetry and Prayer: The Unique Song of the Human Heart

It is written that King David sat on the roof of his palace and at midnight strummed his harp, composing songs, psalms, and laments to God, baring his heart. And, our tradition teaches that when the patriarch Jacob was dying, his sons composed songs about his life, heralding his achievements. The *parashah* in the Torah that speaks of the end of Jacob's life is called *Va-y'chi*, "He lived."

What is it that makes us human? Is it that we must all die, or rather that we all live, achieve, and create and that our achievements endure after our deaths?

"What does God mean to you?" I asked Shirley, one of our group members who had just been diagnosed with Alzheimer's.

"I don't know," she said. "No one has ever asked me that question."

"I am asking you," I said.

"God is doing the right thing," Shirley answered.

I then asked, "How do we know how to do the right thing?"

Evelyn, who has mild cognitive impairment, a possible precursor to Alzheimer's disease, answered, "Sometimes we must do an accounting. Where are we now in our lives? What are our strengths? What are our weaknesses? What can we do to make the world around us better? Even if it is just listening and offering a kind word to those closest to us, sitting at this round table."

Sometimes what we do is intuitive. For instance, Zev Jabotinsky, a poet, journalist, and early Zionist, translated Edgar Allan Poe's poem "The Raven" into Russian, because he wanted to share the poem with the Russian people. Sometimes we feel locked inside ourselves because of circumstance or fear of the approaching end of our life as we know it. In those times, writing poems and prayer may offer help.

One day I asked the group, "How do you write yourself into the world?" We read Psalm 23, "The Lord is my Shepherd, I shall not want."

"What do you want?" I asked.

Shirley, who had just been diagnosed with Alzheimer's disease, answered, "To touch the sky with my fingers, and to hold back the night, because night is when we are taken, when sleep carries us away, when the bogeyman comes out of the closet and captures our spirits."

"Write to God about your fears," I said. "Pretend that you are David the king. It is a warm, summer night, and the wind is blowing. Don't be afraid. The stars will guide you." I played Rabbi Shlomo Carlebach's music and sat down beside them, pens already poised between our fingers. We wrote and wrote. First just words, then sentences. The words flowed like tears, soft and sweet, bitter and sad.

Shirley wrote down her fears, and said she felt forgiven, no longer forsaken. "The world spins and muses," she said, "I'm glad I'm in it."

One day, we read stanzas from *Heart of God* by Rabindranath Tagore, an Indian poet who won the Nobel Prize for Literature in 1913 and who suffered many tragedies in his life, such as the early death of his beloved wife: "I have seen the sea in calm, bearing its immeasurable silence, and in storm, struggling to break open its own mystery of depth."[1] And, we read from Rumi, a thirteenth-century Islamic mystical poet: "All day I think about it, then at night I say it. . . . Where did I come from, and what am I supposed to be doing?"[2] Poetry is a cadence and rhythm of the spirit. Just as King David's poems and prayers, his *t'hillim*, his psalms, have been a salve for people suffering throughout the centuries, so too the act of stringing words into stanzas, of verbalizing our fears into songs, allows us to participate in our healing, to string together the fragments of memory and make sense of the darkness, even the darkness of dementia.

By the Sweat of our Brows Shall We Eat Bread

Just as the Bible teaches that we must work in order to feed, clothe, and shelter ourselves (Genesis 3), similarly active participation in our physical prosperity engenders in us the need to be useful. When we feel ourselves becoming passive, inactive, and even emasculated participants in our own lives, that sense of losing control leaves us empty and depressed. This is the process that many people with dementia experience.

The Bible also teaches that there will come a time when the children will teach the elders, and the elders will learn from the children. People with dementia often feel as if they are losing a part of themselves, and are isolated, but each one of us still has something to contribute to one another, even children and seniors. Walking side by side, and in the act of walking, we become greater than ourselves. Karen Golden, a Jewish storyteller, musician, and teacher in Los Angeles, conducts an enrichment program for homeschooled children. She brought her children to the Jewish Center for an exchange with our seniors. Howard played drums, and the children followed his rhythms. Evelyn sang songs and showed a little girl how to knit. Ya-ae taught them origami. We worked on a mural, old and young, together. We exchanged roles. Sometimes, adults are actually children, who need to be led, guided, and walked through life. Sometimes, we are elders, who teach and cherish our empowerment through guiding others. In each role, we express our godliness through our windows into the Divine; as partners with God, we grow and nurture, and in turn, we are guided, nurtured, and redeemed.

A Visit to the Museum: Revisiting Familiar Pursuits in Unfamiliar Ways

In Genesis, chapter 1, the Bible records that God created the entire world in six days—the physical universe, as well as the emotional and spiritual world. God created a world in which we grow old, our hair becomes gray, and our bodies begin to bow toward the very earth that will eventually accept us back, ashes to ashes, dust to dust. In the meantime, as we journey through this life, we can add texture and substance to our individual, particular memories by exploring familiar realities in unfamiliar ways. Through these windows of opportunity, when memory and consciousness meld, we reach out in yearning for what we failed to do in other phases of our lives or for that which we did not receive in earlier times of our being.

During a recent trip to the Los Angeles County Museum of Art (LACMA), our seniors and children together faced a giant statue of Buddha, centuries old, stoic, unsmiling. "What would you say to the Buddha if you could speak with him?" I asked. This was an outing with the children from Karen Golden's homeschool program. A woman who remains locked in herself because of her dementia, who has seemingly given up on life, reached out her palsied hand to a child next to her. The old woman smiled. A window in her eyes opened.

"I would not speak to the Buddha, to this large mound of stone," the old woman responded. "But I would circle him, in honor of his age, and dance around him. We are the ancient ones of our generation. We are the ones that are left behind. I will not leave him behind. Let us pay homage to him." And so the elders and the children joined hands and we danced the hora around this ancient, imposing figure. And in our dance, we found connectedness, a way to stave off the darkness and reach for the light.

We also did tai chi in LACMA's sculpture garden. We moved with the mobiles. We became the art, our inner rhythms melding with the rhythms around us: the wind, the flowers, the branches rustling. There was Baldessori, a sculpture of a large brain, wall-sized photographs of the ocean on either side, and a screen where we could move, our movements revealed a few minutes after we made them. Words on the wall, reading emotions, creating stories, stepping into landscapes. We become our surroundings, and in the act of becoming and reinterpreting what we knew before, we thereby created new ways of seeing.

Ordinarily, when you view a statue in an art exhibit, you likely would first read the museum curator's explanation of the statue: its origin, how old it is, what materials it was made from, the process of construction. Then, you might examine the statue visually, perhaps marveling at its immensity. Similarly, as you stroll through the sculpture garden, you might remark at the colors of the mobiles, contemplate how they are balanced, and watch as the wind stirs them. Thus, the experience would be passive and intellectual, involving contemplation without interaction.

By contrast, when our group of children and elders with Alzheimer's disease danced the hora around the ancient Buddha and did tai chi in the sculpture garden, we were actively interacting with the art. We incorporated the artistic material into a celebration of body and spirit. In this sense, we were making holistic what we saw and experienced. Fascinatingly, in the museum, we saw how these children and adults are free from intellectualizing their experiences—the children due to their limited, budding intellects, and the elderly on account of their diminishing cognition. With this freedom, they were able to more fully and holistically integrate the art experience.

Mentoring

In the Torah, after he suffered years of imprisonment and then rose to become vizier in Pharoah's court, Joseph gained a special wisdom. When his brothers came to him, seeking grain amid the famine, Joseph taught them to be humble, to be kind, to temper their hatred of him, on account of their love for their father. In Joseph's special way, he was a mentor.

And so, we mentor as well. Adults with dementia who seek to rise beyond their challenges can still follow in the footsteps of Joseph. They can mentor. In our community there are shut-ins who, because of their physical and mental limitations, do not leave their homes. Through their isolation and loneliness, they decline. Nobody hears their remaining wisdom anymore, and nobody remembers their smiles; their memories are left hanging in the air, unharvested.

Edie, one of our group members who is hard of hearing and is confined to a wheelchair, but whose mind is relatively sharp, said, "I want to do something for others. I feel so grateful for each day. Is there anyone we could talk to who has no one to talk to?"

"Yes," I said. "Let's begin with those whom we know of in our community. We can truly be a light among the nations." I have a Japanese friend, Natsu, who is confined to her home because she had back surgery. She loves art and music and is depressed because of her condition. Edie calls her and tells her about her day. They talk about the colors of the sky and what color means to them. They talk about their children, about what it means to get up in the morning, to be a part of each day. They discuss the ordinary things that people say to each other when they are friends.

Unfortunately, in our culture, people with Alzheimer's disease and other cognitive limitations have customarily been compelled to view themselves as only able to be recipients of assistance in various forms. They live in institutions. They attend special programs at community agencies. They have meals prepared for them. They fear being a burden to their families and their communities. Yet, though they may not be able to fully help themselves, that does not preclude their being unable to help others or their being expressive, involved, and creative, even as their cognitive abilities wane. By helping others, such as children or other seniors, they again can feel a valuable sense of self-worth and empowerment. People like Edie, who have always been active and integrated members of their communities, can continue to be, and continue to perceive themselves to be, important communal resources.

Through just being human, even when abilities are diminishing and memories are dimming, we nevertheless can still partner with God, and help make light happen.

And God said, "Let there be light."

10

⚜

From Frustration to Compassion:
A Neurologist's Perspective

RONALD M. ANDIMAN

The elderly couple is sitting before me, as they have every three to four months for the last many years. Abe has a faint smile on his face and seems relaxed. "How are you feeling?" I ask him.

"As long as you can get up in the morning, you've got it made." One might take that as an arguable philosophical position, that for him each day is a blessing. But I know Abe too well for that interpretation; he spends much of his time doing very little. He may be sitting in front of the TV, but he isn't really attending to what is being shown. He does not enjoy sports or politics. He sometimes reads, but he can't tell me anything about what he's read lately. When I press him for the name of any book he's read recently, he says *The Caine Mutiny*. His wife, Shirley, shrugs her shoulders. He may have read that book thirty or forty years ago, but not recently. Yet for Abe each day may indeed be a blessing; who is to judge? The very fact of life is itself a miracle—this cannot be gainsaid. But I also know that Abe is given to speaking aphoristically. At our last visit when I asked how he was feeling, he said, "I feel fine . . . no gain, no strain." His wife, however, is feeling the strain.

"I try to take him out every day," says Shirley. They live in a canyon, on a block without a sidewalk, and the street is steep and curved so that it's dangerous for Abe to walk outside of the home, even if accompanied by his wife, all the more because recently Abe has become unsteady and has had a few falls. Just to get him out of the house, Shirley takes him to lunch every day for a change of scenery. But this has become problematic as well. Abe is impulsive; he'll loudly criticize people before they even do anything wrong. When walking in a crosswalk recently, Abe yelled profanities at a driver thinking that she wouldn't stop in time to let him and Shirley pass, although her driving was unimpeachable and she stopped in plenty of time. "They're anti-Semites," counters Abe to justify his behavior.

"I'm exhausted," says Shirley. Abe frequently awakens in the middle of the night, turning on the lights as he does so. Shirley puts her head under the covers. One night he didn't return to bed for a long time. Shirley got out of bed to find lights on all over the house and everything in disarray. Abe was upset because he couldn't find Shirley, who was in bed, of course, as she always is in the middle of the night. "My son comes once a week to take him out—otherwise I'm 24/7."

Abe thinks the date is February or March 1948; actually, it is April 26, 2011. When I query him about the year, he thinks again and says, "2003." I tell him the actual year and he quips, "What happened to the other seven, the other eight years?" He thinks the Jewish holiday that occurred the week before was, "Rosh HaShanah? . . . Yom Kippur?" He adds 6 + 3 correctly, but says 18 + 16 is "35 or 36." He can remember none of three objects after two or three minutes.

Considering Resources

Is my strength the strength of rock?
Is my flesh bronze?
Truly I cannot help myself;
I have been deprived of resourcefulness.

—Job 6:12–13

I have been a private practice general neurologist in Los Angeles since 1979. The diagnosis and treatment of dementia has always constituted a significant part of my practice. I have seen patients in community hospitals and a large regional academic medical center and have followed them in my offices. Patients have come from all walks of life: the destitute and the wealthy, the self-abusers and those who took exquisite care of their health, those whose premorbid education or intellect was marginal and those who were eminent in their vocations. The dementing processes made victims of all of them, equally.

Over the last thirty years, the science of Alzheimer's disease and related disorders has become more sophisticated. We know more about the microstructure of the disordered neurons and their biochemistry. Diagnostic studies are more precise. There are now medications on the market that offer a modicum of benefit.

But the disease has emotional resonance even for the experienced practitioner. I am no less dispassionate now with my dementia patients than I was years ago, but over the years I have also witnessed the struggles of friends whose lives are stressed by caring for parents of reduced capacity and of old friends who seem to be in the early stages of "losing it." Colleagues a generation older, who used to refer patients to me, later became my patients. Increasingly I recognize that my generation is on the threshold of the appalling geometric increase in Alzheimer's disease incidence that attends the last decades of life.

When people struggle with other life-threatening illnesses that decimate the body, such as cancer, the intellect and the personality are intact enough to allow patients to cope, understand, and at times make peace with their plight. They can recognize the efforts made by loved ones to help comfort and divert them. But those with dementia often have little insight into their plight, and if they do initially, they soon lose that capacity. They have few cognitive or spiritual resources to contribute to their own care and often can't acknowledge the love and caring provided them, except in the most rudimentary ways. Even worse, many demented patients are irascible, angry, cantankerous, argumentative, and physically and verbally aggressive. They may have reversed sleep-wake cycles and keep their families up at night, or they may hallucinate or become delusional.

Frustrations Abound

If I washed with soap,
Cleansed my hands with lye,
You would dip me in muck
Till my clothes would abhor me.
He is not a man, like me, that I can answer Him,
That we can go to law together.
No arbiter is between us
To lay his hand on us both.

—Job 9:30–33

Philip Shore is wheeled into my office by his part-time caregiver. His wife follows. After the exchange of a few pleasantries, the patient recognizes the need to go to the bathroom, and his aide wheels him out. He doesn't always recognize the urge, and his wife is pleased that he still has some level of awareness of bodily function. Over the last few months he has lost his ability to ambulate regularly; when he stands up, his legs shake under him, and he acts as if his legs will give way; he becomes anxious and tries to sit down as soon as possible, even if there is no chair directly behind him. He has no appreciation for what is occurring around him. He doesn't like music and doesn't recognize other people, though he is eating well. When Philip is out of earshot, his wife leans toward my desk. "Is he dying?" she asks. "We've been married for sixty-seven years, and we were together for two years before that. I'm the only one in the world he still knows. If someone else does something for him he thanks me. If he needs to do something and is uncooperative, the attendant says, 'Your wife says you have to take a shower'—then maybe he will."

"Is he dying?" It is a little question from a petite, wrinkled woman. Did I detect a little tremble in her voice, apprehension in her facial expression? What was she really asking? How could she not know?

Her husband has become a faint shadow of himself, but his identity is unchanged. He is still the man who shared all of their experiences as a couple. The elements of his personality and physique that initially attracted her to him cannot be separated from the person he has become. His traits that contributed to keeping their relationship strong over the years are still, in her mind, part of him. But the memories of their life together are hers, alone. Mrs. Shore, I thought to myself, Philip is dying, but what does that mean? We all are in the process of dying from the time we are born.

There is only one way out of this life. But, as Isaac Bashevis Singer once said (though he said it about the Yiddish language), "Between death and dying is a long time." Mrs. Shore was really asking me how much time Philip had left. She needed to prepare herself, to understand some semblance of what she was confronting. For this question there are statistics, but no answers, and no way of predicting the mode of exit.

> Shattered between daybreak and evening,
> Perishing forever, unnoticed.
> Their [tent] cord is pulled up
> And they die, and not with wisdom.
>
> —Job 4:20–21

Encounters, and Not with Wisdom

When I first met Jack Sanford two and a half years ago, he insisted that there was nothing wrong with his memory. He would bring with him a sheaf of papers from his brokerage and insist that I look at them, even when I protested that I didn't want to intrude on his privacy. Thankfully, most of the papers were routine communications, irrelevant to his cause. "Look at this," he would say, tapping at the papers. "If I can do this, there can't be anything wrong with my memory." He says he sold his investments at the beginning of the down market and is "even." At another visit he says, "Even though things were bad for the world they were good for me . . . I have a million dollars in the bank, two million soon . . . I paid off my mortgage." The family had appropriately, some time before, provided his broker with a report from his previous neurologist, documenting his incapability of making rational business decisions. Thus, his broker, who knew Jack for many years, would humor Jack on the phone and deal with his wife on matters of substance.

Nathan's family was less prescient. He had been having difficulty with his memory for some time, but because he lived alone, his daughters were not fully aware of just how much difficulty he was having. When they went on a family vacation, he could not find his bedroom in the rented house. He did not recognize his granddaughter. He would forget where he parked his car and would misplace things. He could not remember a conversation he had with his daughter twelve hours earlier, and he would ask the same questions over and over again. He would have explosive outbursts of temper and would get angry and yell at people for insignificant transgressions. Yet he gave a woman he had just met $500 to "help her out," and then gave her brother $400 to "take the dents out of his car." He was unable to keep track of his bills, so that some were unpaid and others were paid twice. Each month he kept exceeding his budget, and as he was on a small fixed retirement income, this was a problem that was worrisome to his children. Although he was affable and had a hearty sense of humor, Nathan distrusted his daughters and accused them of taking things from him. He would grant them very little access to his financial records and objected to their trying to help him with his bills.

There are several forms of dementia. In Alzheimer's dementia, memory and language are most affected initially, whereas in frontotemporal dementia, also known as Pick's disease, personality and demeanor are affected first. Whereas these categories are organized not only on the basis of clinical presentation but on distinct brain microscopic pathology, each person, in a sense, has his own idiosyncratic form of disease based not only on his subcellular and macroscopic brain dysfunction, but also on his preexisting personality, education, and social milieu.

I remember a patient who divorced his wife of some fifty years and made several terrible financial decisions before his family recognized that these actions were symptoms of dementia, not just an extension of his usual high-handed and imperious personality. The patient had no insight into either his cognitive limitations or the financial and emotional damage he was wreaking on himself and his loved ones. The family had to rely on medicolegal proceedings to prevent him from doing even more damage.

Sensitivity in the Family System

> Isaac said to Jacob, "Come closer that I may feel you my son— whether you are really my son Esau or not."
> So Jacob drew close to his father Isaac, who felt him and wondered, "The voice is the voice of Jacob, yet the hands are the hands of Esau."
> He did not recognize him, because his hands were hairy like those of his brother Esau; and so he blessed him.
> —Genesis 27:21–23

Our patriarch Isaac knew there was a problem. The voice of his son did not match the expected texture of his skin. One would anticipate a thoughtful patriarch to consider and to reason in order to reconcile the contradictory sensory impressions. Isaac did not. Visual loss alone does not explain his behavior. One suspects some sort of cognitive loss in order to explain his impulsivity—patriarchs usually don't toss out blessings willy-nilly—with the legacy of a people at stake. But family relationships also are complicated. Rebecca played favorites; Jacob was immature and self-promoting and lacked moral grounding. And yet it was Isaac's cognitive lapse that allowed an injustice to occur. People with dementia may act irresponsibly and use poor judgment when they lack capacity, and the consequences often are painful. Jacob's relationship with his brother was uneasy forever after. (Of course, the irony is that we owe our nationhood to Jacob's wily and unconscionable behavior.)

In another, modern instance, a highly respected and beloved school principal began to show signs of significant cognitive impairment. Her staff knew something was wrong, but they did not wish to lodge complaints against her with the Board of Education or to embarrass her by being critical and confrontational. Instead, they pitched in and helped with her job until such time as she, herself, realized that she could no longer continue this way. In this case, the patient had the insight to accept help and, with some counseling, knew when it was time to quit.

> He deprives trusty men of speech,
> And takes away the reason of elders.
>
> —Job 12:20

I recently saw an eighty-seven-year-old Persian-American woman who was accompanied by her son and husband. The week before, they reported, she told them that a stranger came into the home, took all of her clothes from the closet, and walked out. On another occasion, when she entered her condominium apartment, she reported seeing a stranger and asked him, "Why are you here?"

The stranger replied, "I had the key and I came inside."

She reported this to her family without any agitation or concern, matter-of-factly. Four months earlier she had asked her son, "Where are the clothes that you brought to the tailor?" when no clothes had been taken to the tailor. She asked her son recently, "Where have you been? You haven't visited me for three weeks." In actuality he had seen her the previous day. On the morning of the medical appointment with me, she asked her husband what day it was; he told her it was Wednesday. A few minutes later she asked, "Is it Saturday?" She had no recollection of having been told it was Wednesday.

As we sit in the office, she says to her family in Farsi, "What is wrong with me?" When I ask her husband to inquire of her if she is experiencing any problems, she says, "No."

Hanokh of Alexandria taught:

> Once there was a stupid man who each morning had a difficult time remembering where he had left his clothes the night before. So one day he got a pencil and a piece of paper and wrote down where he was placing each article of clothing. He placed the note next to his bed and thought to himself, "Tomorrow I will have no trouble finding my clothes!"
>
> He awoke the next morning, quite pleased with himself, took the note, and followed it to the letter, finding each piece of clothing

exactly where he had set it down. Within a short period of time he was fully dressed.

Suddenly he was seized with a terrible thought: "But where am I?" he cried. "Where in the world am I?"

"And so," taught Hanokh of Alexandria, "so it is with us."[1]

If we were all as philosophical as Hanokh, we too could draw homiletic lessons from the small, daily, incessantly mounting agonies of living with a loved one with dementia. The reality, however, is that it is hard to become that dispassionate during this life period of decline and dissolution. Spouses, who are most often the primary caregivers, become cynical, hypercritical, and angry.

Across from me sits a couple. Charlie has a faint smile on his face, and his eyes have a distant look as they wander around the room, inattentive, or seemingly so, to the proceedings in the office. "Look at him," says his wife. "He looks so sweet and gentle. You wouldn't know that he's the meanest sonofabitch alive. Not a kind word ever came out of his mouth. And it's no different now."

Sometimes it's the child who has the major responsibility. Often the parent has been encouraged to move from her home city to that of the child, so that medical care and supervision can be rendered more expeditiously. This works out well until the situation starts to deteriorate. The child's life becomes much more complicated. The parent can't find her car in the parking lot, loses her keys, loses important papers, forgets the conversation about being ready at a certain time for an appointment. She falls, has one too many fender benders, misplaces jewelry and accuses the housekeeper of stealing, and mixes up her medications. It all becomes too much to deal with for a middle-aged child with a job, school-age children, and a husband's needs and who must now learn to accept the peppering of her daily routine with unpredictable emergencies.

A Calculus of Compassion

During encounters in my neurology office, I have seen a daughter refer to her mother coldly as "she," even as her mother sits beside her. "She" is the anonymous third person. The daughter spews a litany of complaints: "She keeps falling, and she won't come to live with me. She won't move into residential care. When I've hired someone to be with her, she fires them. She doesn't see the need and doesn't want to spend the money." The motivation is to keep her mother safe. The tone is one of blame.

On the other hand, I have an elderly patient with very advanced Alzheimer's disease who lives with his unmarried son. His son seems to have infinite patience. He is very solicitous of the old man and engages him in the conversation, repeating to him what I am saying even though the concept is beyond him or the instruction will not be remembered even if it were repeated ten times. The patient is quiet, sometimes smiles, and says little except for sharing social graces at the beginning and the end of the visit.

> R. Abbahu said that when R. Eliezer the Elder was asked by his disciples, "How far should one go in honoring one's father and mother?" he replied, "Go and see what Dama ben Netinah of Ash-kelon did. When his mother who was feebleminded, hit him with her sandal in the presence of the entire council over which he pre-sided, he merely said to her, 'Enough, Mother.' Moreover, when her sandal [with which she was hitting him] fell from her hand, [he picked it up and] handed it back to her, so that she would not get upset."
>
> (*Deuteronomy Rabbah* 1:15; Jerusalem Talmud, *Pei-ah* 1:1, 15c)[2]

Another son takes his father to each of his quarterly appointments with me. The patient had been raised in poverty but was recognized early for his artistic skills and was selected to go to a special technical program where those skills could be developed. In retrospect, he prob-ably had a learning disability, but despite this he distinguished himself in his job as a clothing designer. He had a winning personality and very good business judgment, and he eventually went out on his own and developed and owned several businesses. While the son recounts his father's achievements with pride, the patient says with wonder that he cannot understand how he achieved what he did, given his back-ground. The son is able to remember his father in his loftier days of accomplishment and remains in awe of him even when his speech is impoverished and he has difficulty with everyday activities.

Compassion: The Solution to Frustration

When R. Dimi came [from the Land of Israel], he said: Once, while Dama ben Netinah was seated among the notables of Rome, wearing a silk garment embroidered with gold, his mother came, ripped it off him, struck him on the head, and spat in his face. Yet in no way would he put her to shame.

(Babylonian Talmud, *Kiddushin* 31a)[3]

When R. Eliezer was asked, "How far is a man to go in honoring his father and mother?" he replied, "So far that, should his father take a purse of denars and toss it into the sea in his presence, he would not put him to shame."

(Babylonian Talmud, *Kiddushin* 32a)[4]

There may come a time when unending goodwill, eons of time, and infinitude of love are all frustrated by the progression of disability of the Alzheimer's patient. Yet, if there is a solution, a transformation beyond frustration, even for the physician, it must come in the form of compassion.

The experience of taking care of a person with dementia can be transformative. The husband of a patient asks me to call him later that evening so that he can have a private conversation with me, out of earshot of Yasmin, his wife. He needs advice on how to handle everyday situations. Yasmin asks him to make tea for her and then complains because it isn't being served fast enough. "She has no idea how long things take to do. She's so impatient and yet she is always late. She can never get ready on time. She is very angry all the time. She'll say, 'I told you to get that piece of bread *NOW*,' instead of saying, 'Could you please get it.' She was never like this before." She may ask for something inappropriately expensive. When her husband explains that it is not within their economic means, she gets very angry.

I talk to him about how some of these issues might be handled and about his wife's disease. I ask him to recognize that biologically she's not the same person to whom he's been married all these years. We talk a bit more and then he says, "You know, I think the problem is that up until now I haven't admitted to myself that she's ill."

Not only is the patient transformed by his or her disease, but the caregiver is transformed, too. He may develop insights that he never appreciated under less rigorous conditions. But transformation is a difficult process. To suggest that caring for a person whose intellect and personality are deteriorating daily can be something positive is an attempt at rationalizing or contradicting how obviously awful the situation is—how agonizing, how physically stressful, how depressing, how hopeless it is. Caring for a patient with dementia is not an opportunity for self-improvement; the caregiver is doing what he's doing because he cares.

We tend to search for reasons. What did the patient do wrong to bring this upon him? What did the caregiver do wrong to be saddled with this agonizing responsibility? One cannot help feeling punished. When Job falls prey to one misfortune after another, his friends try to console him by saying that he must accept punishment for his transgressions. But Job protests, "I am blameless. . . . Therefore I say, He destroys the blameless and the guilty" (Job 9:21–23). Job is incensed; he is judged but can't get a fair hearing: "He is not a man, like me, that I can answer Him, that we can go to law together (Job 9:32). But, says Job, "I insist on arguing with God" (Job 13:3). Arguing, searching for meaning, these are part of our tradition. Didn't Abraham argue with God about sparing Sodom if there were even a few innocents living there?

We live in an imperfect world and must try to make the best of it. "Yet who does not live in a world of someone else's making? The trick lies in the attitude one brings to the inevitably compromised life."[5]

When the opportunity arises for me to counsel students or residents who become frustrated when confronted with patients for whom there exists no treatment that will materially affect their condition, I fall back on a little aphorism that I crafted for myself in those situations: "There were doctors before there were cures." I discuss with them what can be done aside from more tests, more drugs, and more physical assaults on the human body. Doctoring is not a technical endeavor; rather, it is a vocation. We are here to serve, both with our understanding of the scientific aspects of disease and with our humanity. We can provide compassion. The thrust toward compassion, I believe, derives from empathy, our ability to identify, not only with the patient but also, especially in the case of the demented patient, with the caregivers. Most physicians who have a modicum of life experience have had encounters with dementia. This is the nidus upon which we build empathy—this and by listening, in psychoanalyst Theodore Reik's terminology, with the "third ear." When we listen deeply, carefully, thoughtfully, actively, we hear the meaning beyond the words that are being said by the patient and by the family. We allow the words to resonate within us and touch us and allow us to respond humanly. The only way of successfully dealing with ineffable tragedy, both on the part of the caregiver and the family, is to do it together. That is the true meaning of compassion. One hopes that the family and patient benefit from our caring and our sensitivity; certainly it will give to the physician the sustenance he or she needs to get through arduous days—a sense of meaning.

> For he who is joined to all the living has something to look forward to.
> —Ecclesiastes 9:4

It is not for physicians to understand the miraculous that is present in that which is human. We can, however, struggle with our patients and their families in awe and in humility.

> Just as you do not know how the lifebreath passes into the limbs within the womb of the pregnant woman, so you cannot foresee the actions of God, who causes all things to happen.
> —Ecclesiastes 11:5

Frustration breeds motivation. The motivation to use what we have learned in dealing with our loved ones can give support and succor to others. Thus, in neurology we have professional meetings dealing with the treatment and management of Alzheimer's and other allied diseases. There are support groups for relatives and recreation groups for patients. Families of patients raise money for research and lobby Congress for more research support. Frustration wedded to motivation may lead to a more justified hopefulness in the possibility of better treatments and, dare we say it, maybe even a cure.

11

⚛︎

Alzheimer's and the Soul: A New Perspective

MICHELE BRAND MEDWIN

Each morning, as part of *Birchot HaShachar*, the morning blessings, Jews offer many different prayers. One prayer always stands
out to me as being different from the others: *Asher Yatzar*. It starts
like any other Jewish prayer—*Baruch atah, Adonai Eloheinu, Mel-
ech haolam*, "Praised are You, Adonai our God, Sovereign of the
universe"—but then the words seem to follow a different path:
". . . who formed the human body with skill, creating the body's
many pathways and openings. . . . If one of them be wrongly opened
or closed, it would be impossible to endure and stand before You."[1]
Having been an eye doctor for thirteen years before I became a
rabbi, this prayer reminds me more of my anatomy classes than my
liturgy classes. While other prayers address souls and peace, Torah
and Israel, this prayer alludes to blood vessels and gastrointestinal
functions. Because of this, however, *Asher Yatzar* may be one of
the most important prayers we offer each day. Most of us take our
health for granted until we no longer have our health. This prayer
reminds us to be thankful that our bodies continue to work properly, day after day.

This prayer has particular meaning for me when I return from visits to my parents. I don't get to see them as often as I would like because I live far away. My father has been struggling with aging issues for the past four or five years. He is wheelchair-bound but also has some cognitive problems, and as his mind slowly changes, the time between my visits can exaggerate these changes for me. He knows who I am and is always happy to see me, but his short-term memory is quite challenged. It is hard for me to see him struggling to remember a conversation we had just moments ago, especially when I reflect on how he used to be. Yes, I am grateful that parts of his body are still working, as the *Asher Yatzar* prayer calls on me to recite. But I am also more and more aware of the parts of my father that no longer work as they once did.

During one visit, I accompanied my mother and father to the doctor's office to consult a new neurologist who was recommended to them. Though I knew that my father's memory was not as it was, this was the first time I heard a doctor say the words "Alzheimer's disease" and associate them with my father.

Medical diagnoses are often difficult to hear and accept. Fortunately, in today's modern medical world, most diagnoses come with cures or helpful treatments. It is possible to have hope that conditions will ameliorate or at least stabilize. For instance, cancer, once the most dreaded and feared diagnosis, no longer always ends in a death sentence. There are many people living for years with a diagnosis of cancer. Advanced medication and surgery along with lifestyle changes can add years to the lives of people diagnosed with heart disease. Both of my parents received such diagnoses. My mother is a breast cancer survivor. Many years ago, when I received her phone call telling me that she had breast cancer, my first reaction was shock and fear. Fortunately, that changed to hope and promise as she was told that the cancer was caught early and the treatments were successful. My father, who had a heart attack at the age of forty-five, is now in his eighties, thanks to medical breakthroughs over the years. But Alzheimer's is not one of those diseases that comes with cures or helpful treatments. Yes, there are some medications that can help delay the advance of the disease, but currently there is no treatment that offers hope for a cure or even for significant improvement. There is only waiting and watching as a person slowly declines.

Being with people who have Alzheimer's disease often is confusing, challenging, and frustrating. In the early or middle stages of the disease, there are times when they seem totally coherent. One can conduct a conversation with them about politics or religion or other areas of interest, and they seem quite "normal." And then, almost without blinking, they suddenly have trouble remembering the answer to the last question they asked, even if the answer was repeated many times. Or, they forget that they even asked the question, and they ask it repeatedly. It is as if they "checked out" for a while when those conversations were under way. It also is hard for them to keep track of other family members who are not present. They can become confused as to family events, such as which grandchildren were married or had graduated from college. Because at times things appear "normal" for such patients, it is easy to forget their limitations, and one may react with frustration or even anger at their inability to respond appropriately to the conversation at hand.

When I am with my father, it is so hard for me to accept that he can be both mentally alert in my presence and then completely gone, within a matter of minutes. It just doesn't make sense to me. I have had in-depth conversations with him about candidates running for political office, and then in the next breath he would ask, "Where are we going for lunch?" even though we just had that conversation five minutes earlier and decided on a restaurant. Once, we were discussing a book he was reading that was written by an author who had a similar upbringing to his own. I was excited that he had the ability to read and remember what he read sufficiently to discuss it. And then in the next sentence he asked, "What are we doing this afternoon?" even though we had decided minutes earlier to take a ride to the beach. I continually want to find some way to return him to that "normal" person that I know he could be, that he just was. And try as I may to be understanding, I often lose patience with him.

After accompanying my parents to the neurologist, I was preparing to leave and return home. While waiting at the airport terminal for my plane to board, I had a chance to rest from the intensity of being with someone who needs so much care and attention. Having some distance from the situation, my emotions turned from frustration and impatience to sadness. A wave of deep sorrow suddenly overcame me as I was forced to acknowledge that the once vibrant, intelligent, and active person I knew and loved was slowly morphing into someone I no longer could recognize at times. I was overwhelmed with a sense of hopelessness. I wondered how much remaining time I had to be with my father until he no longer recognized me. I was searching for explanations, for reasons, for understanding, and, most of all, for comfort.

It is during difficult times like these that I have learned to turn to God for help and solace. My understanding of God has evolved over the past decades. I was an eye doctor before I became a rabbi, and I spent many years studying math and science. My view of God was very logical and orderly at first and needed to "make sense." But during the past ten years I began seeking new ways of connecting to God in a more "spiritual" way. When I released the need to understand God just as I understood science, I was able to find a God who could better provide me with comfort and peace. I began to learn more about the Rabbinic understanding of God, and I read books by authors such as Abraham Joshua Heschel and the Jewish mystics. While waiting at the airport, immersed in my sadness, it dawned on me that in order to be at peace with my father's diagnosis, I had to change my approach. I had to stop thinking of his condition from a medical or logical perspective and see it in a new light. Using a spiritual approach, I realized that there is a different and, for me, a more meaningful way to look at his condition. When my father suddenly "zones out" and is not totally present, I realized that it is helpful to think of the "person" I used to know as not really being "gone," but at that moment, just gone from me. Where does the "person" go, then? I will suggest that his soul visits with God, at least for a while.

According to Rabbinic tradition, the soul is different from the physical body. The midrash explains it this way: "A person's soul is from heaven, and his body is from earth" (*Sifrei Deuteronomy* 306, 132a). This teaching is based on the creation of Adam as described in the Torah. In Genesis we read, "The Eternal God formed man from the dust of the earth. God blew into his nostrils the breath of life, and man became a living being" (Genesis 2:7). Thus, our physical being is connected to the earth, through the dust, and our spiritual being comes from God, via the breath.

There is a beautiful prayer expressing this belief about our souls. This prayer, *Elohai N'shamah*, also is part of *Birchot HaShachar*, the morning blessings, which include *Asher Yatzar*. *Elohai N'shamah* states, "My God, the soul You have given me is pure. . . . You breathed it into me. . . . For as long as my soul is within me, I offer thanks to You."[2] Debbie Friedman (*z˝l*), the celebrated contemporary Jewish singer and songwriter, offered a wonderful way of demonstrating the interweaving of our body and our soul. She sang *Asher Yatzar*, the prayer for our physical health, and *Elohai N'shamah*, the prayer for our spiritual health, together, intertwining the words of both prayers with different, but complementary, melodies.[3]

While in life our physical body and our spiritual soul are fully integrated, that is not so at our death. The Sages believed that when people died, their physical bodies eventually became dust, but their souls continued to live on and join God. From the Talmud we read, "In the world-to-come . . . the righteous sit enthroned, their crowns on their heads, and they enjoy the divine light of the *Shechinah* [a mystical and feminine name for God]" (Babylonian Talmud, *B'rachot* 17a). A modern example expressing this belief is found in a funeral reading from the Reform *Rabbi's Manual*: "The dust returns to the earth as it was; the spirit returns to God who gave it. It is only the house of the spirit which we now lay within the earth; the spirit itself cannot die. Receive in mercy, O God, the soul of our departed. Grant him/her that everlasting peace which You have prepared for us in the world to come."[4]

If we take these ideas, expand on them, and consider them in the context of a person with Alzheimer's disease, we may see this affliction in a new light. The normal understanding of the body and soul in Jewish tradition is that, while together in life, the soul separates from the body at death; we can use this concept and apply it in a slightly different way, to a person with Alzheimer's disease. By seeing the soul and the physical body as already distinct from each other, we can imagine the soul of the afflicted person taking occasional leave of the body, even before physical death. *Olam haba*, the "world-to-come," where souls go after a person dies, is thought of as a place of everlasting peace. Perhaps the soul of the person with Alzheimer's disease also gets frustrated, as we do, by the inability for the person's physical brain to work properly. The soul searches for a way to be at peace. At those moments when our loved ones seem to be "gone and distant," can we imagine their souls taking a short respite, journeying to be with God to seek out a place of peace, even before the physical body ceases to exist?

But how can people continue to live in the earthly realm if their souls are with God? There are three different words in Hebrew for the single English word "soul"—namely, *nefesh*, *ruach*, and *n'shamah*. Post-Rabbinic Jewish philosophers understood the soul of a human being to have three parts, corresponding to these three names. *Nefesh* is the part of our soul that enters us upon our first breath. This is the soul that comes from God and gives us life; therefore, anything that has life has a *nefesh*. *Ruach* is the animal soul. This can be seen as the part of our soul that provides us with our survival instincts—to eat, to sleep, to seek shelter. All animals possess a *ruach* soul. Finally, *n'shamah* is the emotional and intellectual soul—the part of us that makes us "human"—that learns, creates, has feelings and emotions, and forms relationships with other people.

With this understanding of the soul, we can appreciate Alzheimer's disease from a new perspective. When the person we know seems suddenly distant and confused, it might be helpful to think of his "mind" as not just gone, but changing location, from earth to heaven, being with God instead of with us. We can imagine that his *n'shamah*, his intellectual and emotional soul, has temporarily left our loved one's physical body and has journeyed to be with God. Thus even though he doesn't seem to be with us at that moment, we can imagine that he is in a holy place. His *n'shamah* is visiting God, while his *nefesh* and *ruach* remain behind. The person still functions before us, but on a much lower level. The person can still talk, eat, walk, and perform basic functions. With early Alzheimer's disease, we can imagine that it is the *n'shamah* that comes and goes: sometimes it is with us, and sometimes it is with God. His *nefesh* and *ruach* are still with him, continuing to enable him to function physically, even though he doesn't appear to be the person we knew and loved. That aspect of him is missing—no, not missing, just away for a while. When a person reaches the stage of Alzheimer's disease in which he no longer recognizes his loved ones, we can find comfort and seek internal peace by feeling that his *n'shamah* soul, that part of the person that gave him a distinct personality and made him who he was, spends more and more time with God and eventually remains there, even as his body and his two remaining souls are still on earth with us.

It is my dad's *n'shamah* that makes him my father, which includes the characteristics of the relationship we have developed over the years. The *n'shamah* part of his soul is what expresses his love for his family. His *n'shamah* is what gives him his love for Judaism. It is his *n'shamah* that inspired him to teach adult Torah study until he could no longer remember well enough to continue teaching. When my father has difficulties remembering details of his family or is robbed of the ability to teach, it is that very same *n'shamah* that is absent. He still seems to function, however, and can conduct a conversation, but the person who is there is not really my father any longer—at least not the father who was able to do all these things in the past.

My parents are regular Shabbat service attendees and have been since I was a child. I have been with my father at services recently and have noticed that he seems to be at peace while we are there. I believe that this ritual helps him to bring his *n'shamah* back to him and enables him to hold on to it for just a little longer. The familiar melodies and prayers help connect him to the person he used to be before Alzheimer's disease began robbing him of some of his memories. It is as if God hears the prayers and sends his *n'shamah* back, at least for a while longer.

In later stages of Alzheimer's disease, the *ruach*, the animal soul, also starts to take its leave, making it more and more difficult for people to perform the routine tasks of everyday survival. It is harder for them to feed themselves and care for their own physical needs.

This can cause much strain on family members and caregivers. Yet, we can try to find comfort in a spiritual approach to the disease if we imagine the *ruach*—the animal soul—joining the *n'shamah* and spending more and more time, elsewhere, with God. Eventually only the *nefesh*, the breath in them, remains, until that too finally departs to be with God at death. When most people die, all parts of the soul leave simultaneously and depart to be with God. In the regression of one with Alzheimer's disease, we can envision the soul breaking into its three disparate parts, with each segment of the soul departing separately and independently, often periodically journeying back and forth between heaven and earth before remaining permanently with God. For me, believing that my father's *n'shamah* is with God when he doesn't seem to be aware of his surroundings, when he is confused and disoriented, has become a source of comfort to me and helps give me patience when he repeats the same question for the tenth time.

Prayer has always been a means to help me get through difficult times. In keeping with Reform Jewish tradition, sometimes making a few changes in the texts of the prayers can add another dimension to a particular prayer, endowing it with additional, new meaning. As I reread some of the morning blessings, I rediscovered a prayer that I have recited often, but which took on new meaning after my visit with my father, when I learned to see his Alzheimer's disease in this new light:

> *Modeh/modah⁵ ani l'fanecha, Melech chai v'kayam,*
> *she-hechezarta bi nishmati b'chemlah,*
> *rabbah emunatecha.*

> I offer thanks to You, ever-living Sovereign,
> that You have returned my soul to me in mercy:
> How great is Your trust.⁶

When this prayer was written by the Rabbinic Sages, it was believed that one's soul left the body to be with God during sleep and then it returned to the body as the person awoke in the morning. It was a prayer thanking God for allowing us to reawaken each morning, with our souls returned to us. Seeing a person with Alzheimer's disease as a body with a multifaceted soul, this prayer can be understood anew. We envision the soul journeying to sojourn with God, not during sleep, but during those times when the person is physically present, but cognitively absent.

I have rewritten this prayer to be recited by loved ones of a person with Alzheimer's disease (changes are in capital letters). If you were offering this prayer for a man you would say:

> *Modeh ani l'fanecha, Melech chai v'kayam,*
> *she-hechezarta BO NISHMATO BAZ'MAN HAZEH, b'chemla,*
> *rabbah emunatecha.*

> I offer thanks to You, ever-living Sovereign,
> that You have restored HIS *N'SHAMAH* TO HIM, AT THIS
> MOMENT, in mercy:
> How great is Your trust.

If you were offering this prayer for a woman you would say:

> *Modah ani l'fanecha, Melech chai v'kayam,*
> *she-hechezarta BA NISHMATA, BAZ'MAN HAZEH, b'chemla,*
> *rabbah emunatecha.*

> I offer thanks to You, ever-living Sovereign,
> that you have restored HER *N'SHAMAH* TO HER, AT THIS
> MOMENT, in mercy:
> How great is Your trust.

Dad, I offer this prayer for you.

12

❧

Memory Is Incumbent upon the Jew:
But What about My Mother's Dementia?

ELYSE GOLDSTEIN

I loved the goofy movie *50 First Dates*, with Adam Sandler. In this film, Sandler plays Henry Roth, a veterinarian living in Hawaii who leaves the playboy life behind after he falls for a beautiful woman named Lucy, although there's a catch: Lucy suffers from short-term memory loss sustained after a terrible car accident. Since she can never remember meeting him, Henry has to romance Lucy every single day and hope that she falls for him again and again. Therefore, every day is a new adventure, even if they repeat the same pattern over and over again; even if they go to the same diner and say the same sentences repeatedly, it is exciting, fresh, and novel each time for Henry. It is never boring to eat the same waffles or sing the same song or laugh at the same joke when you are in love. *50 First Dates* has a magical happy ending. The couple gets married, and Henry makes Lucy a videotape that she watches every morning to remind her of who he is—and who she is—and they live happily ever after. Each morning begins a new adventure with new love for a new partner.

The movie left me so optimistic: perhaps it is possible to see my mother's dementia as a new adventure every day! Maybe I can make her a videotape of who I am that she can watch before my visits! Life isn't Hollywood, though; it is more like a reality TV show. You get put into awkward situations like in the old *Candid Camera* show: your mother doesn't recognize her own grandchild, and you have to "cover" for her or assure your child that her grandma still loves her. The "audience" (your family, the nursing home staff, other residents) watch as you wriggle through. You get a few laughs. Everyone else can change the channel, but you have to star in the next episode over and over again. It is painful, truly painful.

Unlike the cute premise of *50 First Dates*, every day is not a new beginning for my mother, although on the surface it could be seen as such. Every *Kol Nidrei* when she is not in her usual seat, front row, looking up at the bimah at me and smiling with *nachus*, is not a sweet Hollywood moment. When I took the shofar to her nursing home and blew it for her, she covered her ears and said, "Oh, loud."

Her hearing is failing, and her sight is bad. She keeps forgetting to put on her glasses anyway, so life is even more of a blur than it is already because of her fading memory. She is still here spiritually. I feel her *n'shamah*—her soul—shining through the sometimes vacant moments, her smile still lighting up the room when I walk in, even if she isn't 100 percent sure of why I am there or who is that nice man with me. She does not know that I moved to a new house, because the anxiety it would cause her, the insecurity of not understanding where I now live, is not worth it. She does not know the name of her nursing home, and she thinks she just moved there, even though she's been there for three years. Yet, when she smiles, I still see my mother as she once was, a long time ago.

When my mother smiles, I see her familiar dimples. When she smiles, I see the Terry "then" who once was the executive director of the National Federation of Temple Youth. I see her ordering rabbis around, I see her singing in a song session, I see her holding court while hosting her famous *Oneg Shabbat* from the front porch of her faculty cabin at Kutz Camp in Warwick, New York. When I realize that I, too, have been "vacant" during the past few moments of reminiscing, I force myself to see the "now" Terry, confined to a wheelchair, struggling to put together a full sentence, and being fed by a nurse. I see that she is still my mother, but she has also become my child. It is a cruel reversal of caregiving. A memory is a terrible thing to lose.

Our family has come to accept it with only a small degree of equanimity. My children don't really want to visit, but they visit if I ask them to do so. I don't look forward to the nursing home seder or Chanukah party, where she sits overwhelmed, but I go anyway. It is what it is, and it's not getting better. There are even some advantages to my mom's lack of memory, we discovered. No use worrying about the time I was a little short-tempered with her, because she won't remember it and it doesn't bother her. No use aggravating myself that she lost her bracelet, because she doesn't remember ever having it and she's not upset that it's gone. She's happy with little things for a very short while: going out for Chinese food means more than the actual reason we're going out, which she can't remember, whether it is someone's birthday, or Mother's Day, or Chanukah. She doesn't remember the meaning of Rosh HaShanah, so she doesn't agonize about her shortcomings or failures or the need to do better, or what she should wear to services, or even if she should go. Each day is just each day, and she takes it as it comes. There are some advantages to not having short-term memory. It is like the man who goes to the doctor, and the doctor tells him he has both cancer and Alzheimer's. The man pauses for a moment and says brightly, "Well at least I don't have cancer!" My mother tends to look on the bright side. When I remind her that she is eighty-eight years old she says, "Well, at least I'm not over eighty. . . ."

But a memory is a terrible thing to lose. And I, as a Jew, live and breathe in the world of memory. The Jews are a people of memory. In his book *Zakhor: Jewish History and Jewish Memory*, historian Yosef Hayim Yerushalmi writes, "Only in Israel . . . is the injunction to remember felt as a religious imperative to an entire people."[1] Memory is incumbent upon the Jew. It is a commandment: Remember! We must remember that we were slaves in Egypt; we must remember the Sabbath to keep it holy; we must remember our enemies, like Amalek.

"Remember . . . don't forget!" (Deuteronomy 25:17–19). Interestingly, here the Torah uses a double imperative, as if it is fearful that remembering is not enough, as if "not forgetting" is necessary too. Is this a different action, to "not forget"? Is it not the same as "remembering"? I am not sure, but when I visit my mother I feel somehow that she is actively forgetting, a little more each day. The Hebrew root *zachor*, "remember," appears 169 times in the *Tanach*, the Hebrew Bible, and we could argue that the English translation of *zachor* as "remember" is too small in scope; "remember" fails to capture the grandness of the imperative, "*Zachor!*" The word *zachor* implies a level of action: not just remembering, but also not forgetting, as in Moses' brilliant final oration in Deuteronomy when he cries out, "O Israel, remember and do not forget!" It is a kind of holy refrain, like a parent's cry, "Do not cast me off in old age; when my strength fails, do not forsake me" (Psalm 71:9).

Memory is incumbent upon the Jew because memory is the beginning of action. Moses begs the people not only to remember, but to act so that the work he started is someday finished. It's not enough to sing with Barbra Streisand about "misty water-colored memories of the way we were," without having a map for the way we will be. Memory is incumbent upon the Jew, but it is of no value if it doesn't move us from the past into the future. For instance, we welcome strangers because we remember what it was like to be strangers in Egypt.

Memory is incumbent upon the Jew, but it is also incumbent upon God. In the Book of Exodus, Moses saves the day for the Jewish people not by engaging in grand argument, but rather when he jogs divine memory. He challenges God, "Remember Abraham, Isaac, and Jacob!" (Exodus 32:13). The *Zohar*, the mystic book of Kabbalah, teaches, "And God remembered the covenant with Abraham, with Isaac and with Jacob. Truly this remembrance is the foundation and root of the whole Torah and the basis of all the commandments and of the real faith of Israel" (Soncino *Zohar*, *Sh'mot* 2:38a).[5] Rosh HaShanah is called *Zichron* in Leviticus 23:24, "the day of memory," because we ask God to remember us, as we say in the High Holy Day *Amidah*: *Zochreinu l'chayim*, "Remember us unto life." Even if we do not remember who we are, from where we came, or why we say the prayer, still we ask God to remember *for us*. It is as if being remembered will help us to remember.

So what are we to remember? Ancient facts and figures, seas parting and plagues visited, and kings of yesteryear? The way we were back in the shtetl? No. We may think we should remember our history, but history is what happened, and memory is what it means to us. Remembering Jewish history is of value only if it helps us to reconnect to what it means to be a Jew in the present tense, in the present time and space we occupy. It makes sense to go backward only to refashion what we once knew. However, in truth, we can't really remember our history, because at best what we have of it is a reconstruction anyway. "Memory is a complicated thing, a relative to truth, but not its twin," writes Barbara Kingsolver in her book *Animal Dreams*.[2]

We remember the past as we think it was, but not necessarily as it actually was. Thus, when we celebrate a past, we celebrate *what we think that past might have been*, rather than what we know for sure it was. In fact, we might actually be celebrating what that past *ought to have been*. I realize that when I remember my mother doing Israeli dancing with me at camp many years ago, very possibly I am conjuring a scene that may never have really happened as I picture it. When I reconstruct the memory of my mom at her office desk working, I am remembering a productive, busy, and smart woman who ran a whole organizational department. Perhaps in reality, however, she was frustrated, made to feel inadequate, unsure of herself, unskilled. But that is not the workday I am remembering at all. Yerushalmi writes:

> What is Jewish memory, after all, but deliberately constructed mythical nostalgia that binds one to a past even in radically reinterpreting that past? Jewish memory scoffs at the definition of memory as a first-order photographic capture of experience lived. Instead, Jewish tradition ironically celebrates temporal distance from the actual event being remembered, translating the event into ritual, nostalgia, and myth. Jewish memory is not made more correct by its historical accuracy. This translation of event to practice bridges the chasm of past and future, and renders a specific historical event into an ongoing event of significance.[3]

In other words, the real faith of Israel is our ability to take a memory and either translate it into a ritual that has everlasting value, whether or not the specific, remembered event actually happened precisely, or use the memory to trigger reflection, values, and ethics that also bear everlasting value irrespective of their actual historicity.

Judaism lives in the present when it radically reinterprets its past—without losing its memory. We radically refashioned our memory of what the Temple in Jerusalem was, while ensuring its continued role in Jewish life, when we invented the synagogue. We radically refashioned our memory of what the ancient nation of Israel was, thus ensuring its continuity, when the modern State of Israel was born in 1948 as a democracy. As we refashion Shabbat, the holidays, and the "look" of the Jewish home, we both hold our memories of Shabbat in perpetuity and also free Shabbat from being "stuck" forever in one mold.

Put personally, it doesn't matter who my mother was; it matters who I remember she was. This may be a radical reinterpretation of the past, but it helps me live in the present. While I am struggling with her inabilities now, I do not need to remember her inabilities of the past. If reconstructing that memory of her *Oneg Shabbat* at camp does not include the petty fights or politics of that summer but is cast in a pleasant sepia tone of a romanticized past, that beauty helps me now retain the image of her as beautiful. Even as she cannot today choose a necklace, I remember her dazzling jewelry chest from the past, and I do not focus on the rusted pieces. Thus, I am less upset when she cannot find the new pin I just brought her from Israel.

Jonathan Safran Foer, in his book *Everything Is Illuminated*, puts it beautifully when he writes:

> Touch, taste, sight, smell, hearing, memory . . . for Jews memory is no less primary than the prick of a pin, or its silver glimmer, or the taste of the blood it pulls from the finger. The Jew is pricked by a pin and remembers other pins. It is only by tracing the pin-prick back to other pinpricks—when his mother tried to fix his sleeve while his arm was still in it, when his grandfather's fingers fell asleep while stroking his great grandfather's damp forehead,

when Abraham tested the knife point to be sure Isaac would feel
no pain—that the Jew is able to know why it hurts. When a Jew
encounters a pin, he asks: What does it remember like?[5]

"What does it remember like?" is not the question for a lot of Jews
today. Collective memory doesn't work for our generation whose
grandparents don't speak Yiddish, whose parents know little of Jewish tradition or culture, whose kids are tied with the thinnest of thread
to the idea that they are Jewish. It doesn't work for converts to Judaism, who didn't "stand at Sinai" but entered on their own, devoid of
Jewish nostalgia from not having grown up Jewish. It doesn't work for
the Jew from a small town, the Jew isolated, the Jew on the margins
whose "amen" is not heard, who does not remember the other pin-
pricks of his or her history. A central question for Jews today is this:
In a world in which so many people live largely only in the present,
how capable are we of feeling a common bond with other Jews? Is
common memory a factor anymore in the development of a mutual
connection? With little or no collective memory anymore, and little
individual memory, we suffer from Jewish amnesia.

We live in a society afflicted with collective amnesia, so we're not
alone. Our culture is too impatient to dwell on the past; we chalk it
up as "outdated." It takes less than two years for new technology to
become obsolete. Use it up quickly, get rid of it, and then move on. We
are a culture of "and next up . . ." in which newscasters move quickly
from a terrible news story to a sweet "human interest" segment or a
commercial break. We live, like a woman with no memory, only in this
moment. Look at our treatment of the environment: if it is good now,
we use it now with little regard for what it will mean tomorrow. Dar-
fur, the Sudan, Bosnia: we are doomed, as Professor George Santayana
prophesied, to repeat history because we do not learn from it, because
we have forgotten. Sometimes we all act like aging parents with little
memory left.

It is incumbent upon the Jew to remember. That is true. But I am
praying for something else. I am praying to be remembered, to live in
such a way so as to leave a legacy. Let the world be better because I

have been in it. To be remembered is to not disappear. To be remembered is to be validated. To be remembered is to be present even when absent. To be remembered is to be re-membered: to be a member once again of community and context. I am praying for my mother to be remembered, because that is all she can have now: to be re-membered into my life and my family, to be treasured for her legacy and to be loved for her absence as much as for her presence.

In *50 First Dates*, even love cannot reverse a brain injury, and Lucy doesn't get her short-term memory back; neither will my mom. "What does it remember like?" I ask myself when I leave the nursing home after a visit. I have decided, taken an oath, that my mom will be remembered even if she doesn't remember. To remember and to be remembered are precious gifts, but they are different gifts. The first we cannot control; the brain will do its own thing regardless of what we want. Memories fade away and are gone. They fade because, in the words of the Psalmist, "We fly away" (Psalm 90:10). No matter how many mementos and snapshots we paste into scrapbooks and photo albums, as much as we vow to "never forget," eventually, one way or another, we do. But to be remembered is altogether possible. It is why we say *Yizkor*. It is why we chant *Avinu Malkeinu* and ask God with all our rational and modern hearts to remember us in the Book of Life. Memory is where we place our future as Jews and our hope as human beings.

PART III

Moving On

13

❧

Care at Home or Care in a Home?

Toby F. Laping

My beloved cousin recently died of Alzheimer's disease at age eighty. Arnold had been a brilliant man, a top lawyer with astute judgment. He was used to being in control, and he was accustomed to having a staff who did his bidding. This was a man for whom seemingly incomprehensible situations were challenges to be understood and then made rational.

When Arnold received his Alzheimer's diagnosis, he fought against it with vigor even as it quickly overwhelmed his brain. His underlying personality remained intact, and he behaved just as we would have expected of a healthier Arnold. He railed against the inevitable limitations on his freedom, and he fought the newly imposed structures that helped him continue to function. He constantly pulled apart his home trying to make sense of what his brain couldn't absorb; he tore apart books, he moved furniture, he searched endlessly for unknown objects that would help him understand. Ultimately his wife, Sue, reluctantly agreed with me that Arnold would be better served in a nursing home, because he needed the structure of a facility, as well as the simpler, more basic environment of a nursing home. I also hoped that away from his home, he would abandon his futile, frustrating, and frantic efforts to create a more comprehensible world.

Thankfully, placement worked for him. Arn settled into an institutional routine that seemed to give him some measure of comfort. He loved Sue's daily visits, and when she left for the night, he was generally accepting of the required care. For him, moving out of the house was the right choice.

We were lucky with Arn. Our instincts worked. That doesn't always happen.

For many years, my professional life has been spent as a geriatric care manager. Families come to me and my professional firm in Buffalo, New York, for consultative advice on how to deal with their relatives when they have problems related to aging. They want to know how to manage illnesses, where they can find help and how to pay for it, whether it's okay to get angry and frustrated, and how much of themselves to surrender in trying to make life better for their relative. Typically, I work to develop a clear picture of the family unit, including personal information about how the family functions, relationships between family members, and their financial life, including priorities for spending money. I need to understand who has been the decision maker and whether decisions affecting family members are made unilaterally or by negotiations. I determine whether the family unit is comfortable spending money on caregiving, whether the children are going to provide emotional and/ or financial support, and if so, whether that support will be given grudgingly or willingly. Begrudged support may be short-lived and unreliable. I need to determine whether the family that is reasonably stable financially will jeopardize its lifestyle in order to care for its loved one at home or whether to look to government funding or entitlements in order to best preserve resources. In other words, I develop a fairly complete picture of the family and then design and implement the most appropriate, viable road map for the immediate, intermediate, and long-term future. Usually there also is the question, either spoken or implied, "Should we keep him home?" or phrased differently, "Does she belong in an institution?" They ask me the same questions Sue and I asked ourselves about Arnold, and they hope for a clear, indisputable answer, even when one doesn't exist.

Families, including even those with the brightest and most rational minds, search for the magic potion that will make life easier, that will let them know what to do, and that will help the person with dementia to understand what's happening and to know that he's still loved. At the same time, they commonly want the person to grasp the need to try harder to be what he used to be. And, they want an answer to the question of why the patient won't remember. They'll remind the patient that he's been told to go to the toilet before he's panicky because he's soiled his pants; they'll remind the patient that she needs to take her medications at the same time each day or they'll not give the benefits they promise. And then, families feel guilty when they remember that the patient can't remember. It isn't that she doesn't want to cooperate, but that she just is not able. And that's when they search for some solution—some way to deal with this—so that everyone isn't so tired and frustrated and short-tempered all the time. And I think to myself, "Welcome to the awful world of Alzheimer's, where there's no good answer and every solution has a downside." But then I give the more gentle response, "Let's look at the options and see what fits your family best. And, you're doing as well as you could possibly do, so let's try to figure this out without the guilt you're clearly feeling."

That's when I so often think of those wonderful lines of the Mishnah in *Pirkei Avot*, from the ancient sage, Hillel:

> If I am not for myself, who will be for me?
> If I am for myself alone, what am I?
> And if not now, when?
>
> —*Pirkei Avot* 1:14

Those sacred verses articulate and make sense of the conflicts that families feel. They give permission to caregivers to pay attention to their own needs. Indeed, it's more than acceptable; it's essential to do so before we can help others. Hillel's first question, "If I am not for myself, who will be for me?" reminds us to be sensitive to ourselves and our own needs. After that, we're reminded that we must also attend to the needs of our patients: "If I am for myself alone, what am I?" And then, if those needs are in conflict, adjustments must be made promptly: "And if not now, when?"

In the slow, grinding deterioration that typifies Alzheimer's disease, it becomes clear who holds the power to make decisions and how the balance of power in families often changes with the progression of the disease. I see love stories that flourished for decades but are now at risk of deteriorating into recriminations or fatigue. I also see relationships that had long been mediocre at best now begin to flourish with an awareness of how much the caregiving partner is needed and how desperately the demented partner depends upon the spouse. And sometimes, I see those families for whom caregiving—whether directly or by paid caregivers—is simply love and what one does for one's beloved. It is at such times that I am deeply touched by the depth of caring of which we are capable.

Sometimes, families come to me convinced that they will keep their demented loved one living at home, and they imagine that that person will remain stable, as he is now. But, he will not remain stable, neither functionally nor emotionally; the disease process will take its toll. Families will soon enough face the reality that the essence of their loved one is no longer present and that their loved one may need more, or something different, from that which they can provide.

Imagine the guilt that could be instantly absolved if there was an absolute answer to the question of whether and when a loved one should be placed in an institution. Of course, there is no universal, correct answer, and there is no one-size-fits-all, generic formula for determining when to institutionalize a person with Alzheimer's disease. Instead, the answer is a process of soul-searching that takes into account relationships from prior to the onset of the illness, the emotional tolerance of caregivers, the personality of the ill person, and even such a basic concern as money.

Our tradition gives us some guidance. In his volume *The Book of Jewish Values*, Rabbi Joseph Telushkin quotes Maimonides: "If one's father or mother becomes mentally disordered, [the child] should try to indulge the vagaries of the stricken parent, until he [or she] is pitied by God (and dies). But if he finds he cannot endure the situation because of the parent's madness, let him leave and go away, and appoint others to care for the parent's property."[1] Telushkin contemporizes this thought by urging that children should do their best to care for parents, whether on their own or with outside help. He writes, "As for sending a parent to live in an old age home, this should be a final step, never a first one."[2]

Some years ago, I knew a remarkable gentleman named Bill. He and his wife, Ruth, had been married for decades and were still deeply in love. She developed Alzheimer's disease, and even as she deteriorated rapidly, he continued to treat her with the same gentleness and respect that he had always shown her. Ultimately, he was forced to move her to a nursing home, because she required two helpers for some of her activities of daily living. Bill had no financial resources to hire private help, and Medicaid would neither provide enough hours of help at home nor pay for two aides in the house. Bill selected a nursing home near his house so that he could visit Ruth daily. He brought his lunch from home and had lunch with his wife every day, and frequently he stayed at the nursing home for dinner. He went with her to every activity run by the facility. Whenever the larger community had a parade or carnival or other fun event, Bill picked up Ruth at the institution, and they went together to the event. Her life was as rich and as full as she could absorb, and Bill was intimately involved in Ruth's life. She felt safe and cherished, and her contented demeanor reflected that.

I used to think that Bill was painfully demanding of himself, but over the years I came to understand that this wasn't the case, at all. He acted out of love and devotion, and it would have been excruciating for him to have stayed away. As well, Bill knew that the quality of Ruth's life was in his hands. I have learned that the Jewish ideal of true love is giving, as opposed to loving with a goal of being loved in return, and Bill's selfless love epitomized that ideal. Ruth wasn't able to tell him he was loved; she had already lost the gift of language, and she often didn't even give him a welcoming or loving smile. Still, Bill continued in his faithful role of husband, and perhaps inadvertently and surely without premeditation, Bill received immense satisfaction. "If I am not for myself, who will be for me?" Bill was not conflicted, though he was not acting for himself.

For all sorts of reasons, families and spouses decide how much of themselves will be dedicated to the caregiving role. Ironically, the same decision—whether to keep someone in the home or to find institutional placement—may come from the most base or the most deeply caring motivations. A family may make a loving, heartfelt review of options, or a family may decide on the same course of action based on anger and a desire to punish. Is the spouse who previously felt subservient now suddenly empowered? Is the spouse who felt cheated in the marriage now the one who decides where the demented partner should live? Or, is the caregiving spouse the one whose satisfaction in life comes from caring for others and being needed? Is the caregiving spouse willing to provide whatever environment allows her loved one to feel safe? "If I am for myself alone, what am I?"

The question of whether a loved one should be placed in an institution or kept at home requires an examination of the options as well as the motivations that inform decision making. Soul-searching is never easy, and reviewing the nature of the relationship prior to the onset of the illness can be disconcerting but can help explain why we make the decisions we make. Further, such soul-searching can help ensure the best possible balance between conflicting needs—being for ourselves and the needs of the Alzheimer's patient—or not being for ourselves alone.

Barbara was always a timid person who looked to her husband, Joe, for clues about how to behave, for guidance about what she should like and what she should do, and for validation of her actions. Joe had learned over the years that Barbara needed his approval in even the most mundane decisions in order to feel secure. Thus, he thought nothing of it when she became increasingly unable to make decisions, even about such petty and insignificant things as what blouse to wear or how to prepare dinner. Actually, it wasn't until Barbara's doctor noticed her significantly increased difficulty recalling recent events that Joe began to consider the extreme extent to which Barbara was now depending upon him, well beyond the dependency that she had shown as recently as two years earlier. Barbara was diagnosed with Alzheimer's-type dementia, but she and Joe continued to live as they had previously. Joe was used to making decisions, and he saw their present situation as more extreme, but not substantially different, from the way that they had always lived. Joe occasionally felt put upon, but he recognized that Barbara's personality was now just an exaggeration of what it had always been, and he was willing to continue in his role of protector and director. For Joe, keeping his wife at home was no big deal, and she lived there until her death.

Joe was unique. Almost always, there is increased isolation and stress for everyone in an Alzheimer's family, including both the patient and those who love him. Even despite that increased stress, however, family members can and sometimes do grow in their abilities to care and to help the patient feel cherished. Joe never felt he was doing anything special, but he surely was. It is deeply gratifying to hear and see expressions of love, protectiveness, and sensitivity toward a patient who cannot respond and who cannot return caring in kind. Watching families develop their abilities to express love so openly and unabashedly can be remarkable, and even startling, particularly if they had previously been taciturn and reserved.

The brilliant twentieth-century philosopher Martin Buber described relationships as largely "I-It." These are functional, surface relationships that may have emotional content and be perfectly pleasant, but are relationships in which we rarely expose ourselves emotionally or open ourselves to hearing or caring for the deepest feelings of others. Even more rarely, when we are sufficiently receptive, we engage in "I-Thou" relationships, in which we allow the full depth of emotional being to show, and we respond to that exposure in someone else. I-Thou moments become sacred occasions, and it is as though God requires us to have these moments in order for God to become actualized in our lives. I sometimes understand growth in expressing love as a beautiful image of Martin Buber's sacred I-Thou relationship, although Buber imagined an emotional reciprocity that can unlikely exist in the person with dementia. Still, when families tell a patient how deeply he's loved and how much he's needed, with all the emotional exposure that implies, such love is essentially selfless. The only apparent benefit for the caregiver is knowing that her loved one feels cherished in that moment; the caregiver is reflecting the fullness and holiness, reaching into the depths of the person who is cared for, of Buber's I relating to the Thou.

The perspective of families, the balance in relationships, and the neediness of the patient all affect how we respond to a patient with Alzheimer's and help determine how much of ourselves might be engaged in the caregiving process without ourselves becoming unbalanced. Sometimes, the caregiver becomes more loving and demonstrative once someone else has taken over the nitty-gritty, sometimes frustrating details of caregiving.

> If I am not for myself, who will be for me?
> If I am for myself alone, what am I?
> And if not now, when?

Sue is now seventy-nine. Her husband of fifty-six years, Mark, died a few years ago following a dementia that was remarkably stable for several years, after which he had a precipitous decline and died within six months. Mark had been a strong personality whose wishes had ruled the family. Three years earlier, Mark decided that he and his wife would sell their home and move to an elegant assisted-living facility. Sue opposed the move. She loved her home, her children lived within a mile of them, and she had sufficient help to maintain the house easily. Nevertheless, unilaterally Mark decided on this move, and he selected a facility approximately twenty-five miles from their home. Their house was put on the market and sold quickly, packers and movers were lined up, and a house sale dealt with the multitude of belongings that would never fit into the new assisted-living unit.

Sue acquiesced in order to please her husband. She was aware that he had been diagnosed with dementia, but facing that, as well, was too painful, and she dismissed it to the back of her mind. The couple moved, and within two months of the move, Mark's previously diagnosed Alzheimer's became pronounced. Symptoms probably had been there previously, but now, in an unfamiliar environment and without a fixed routine, those symptoms were visible and disturbing. Sue increasingly found herself acting as the full-time caregiver for a husband who rapidly lost his ability to reach out and interact socially or to make rational decisions. Mark, who had been so controlling, was sufficiently aware of events and became furious when he could not control his disease.

Mark quickly became wholly dependent on Sue, and when she tried once or twice to hire help so she could have a break from caregiving, Mark's anger became intense and Sue relented. Ultimately, Mark became so severely demented that he needed nursing home placement, but by that time, Sue was exhausted and angry and without a nearby support system. Her new neighbors long ago gave up trying to reach out to her, and as often happens, they now kept even greater distance lest they be associated with someone with dementia. Sue's life lost its quality, and she was unable to retrieve it. "What am I?"

I suspect that Sue had been angry with Mark for years because of his disdain for her preferences and decisions, but now that he was no longer able to override her, she was in charge and she wanted to punish him. He was admitted to a nursing home, and once that happened, Sue rarely visited him. When he died, she breathed a sigh of relief that she could finally enjoy her life without his condemnation of her decisions. It was terribly sad, but consistent with the way they had lived their married lives.

Should Sue have insisted on remaining in her home? Quite possibly she should have, but she did not have the strength to do so. Should Mark have been more willing to accommodate Sue's desires? The reasonable answer is, of course, but it did not happen. Should he be blamed if she didn't demand that her wishes be heard and addressed? Perhaps blame is irrelevant; the situation had lingered for years, even decades, without either party taking steps to change things. Should Sue have been so willing to be the sole and full-time caregiver, when it was obvious that there was sufficient money to hire help? In observing the decisions and the relationship, important dynamics emerged and sadly buried both members of this couple.

It is clear that being so self-sacrificing as to neglect one's own needs does oneself an injustice. "If I am not for myself, who will be for me?" Self-sacrifice also fed Sue's anger as the subservient partner, and that is damaging to any relationship, as well as to one's individual psyche. The anger of over-sacrificing for a spouse with Alzheimer's disease, in this case, eats one away, and it can cause depression, hostility, and endless poor and damaging decisions.

Those of us who work with elderly couples with an ill partner often see the caregiving spouse sadly die before the person for whom they're caring. Sometimes—though not always—it is because the selfless care-givers have forgotten that they must care for themselves before they can care for others. As well, we've seen children's marriages founder because an adult child cannot separate from the endless needs of an ill, otherwise lonely parent.

I recently worked with a couple, Alan and Ellen. Alan developed a quickly progressing form of Alzheimer's, and Ellen wisely hired help to be with Alan from morning until evening, when she returned home and could assume responsibility. This put a painful strain on their budget, but Ellen felt it was money well spent. One evening while she was making dinner, Ellen was paying attention to her cooking and didn't realize that Alan was absent. He had managed to disable the house alarm system that Ellen used in order to know that Alan was safely in the house. He used the same code the family had used for many years. His memory of things long ago was still intact, although he had no recall of recent events; his mind couldn't encode new memories, but he could retrieve those old numbers.

Alan slipped out of the house and wandered around the neighborhood for about half an hour. Ellen called the police, desperate for help and panicked about Alan's whereabouts. Alan was found shortly thereafter, safely wandering the sidewalk near his house and was returned home, though the police officer gave Ellen a stern warning to be a better caregiver in the future. On edge even before this incident because of her husband's condition, Ellen was so distraught over the situation and by the inappropriate lecture by the policeman, that it was clear that she couldn't continue with things as they were. It was time to put her husband in a facility where she could visit him, and she could be a better, calmer, more loving wife because others would be responsible for Alan's safety.

Ellen and I discussed this at length. I was seriously concerned for Ellen's health and her stress level. Her first response was that Alan shouldn't be institutionalized on account of her stress, but she was objective enough to see that no one was well served as things stood. Her husband was at risk, and she was frantic. And, she was able to see that Alan was no longer deriving pleasure from his familiar surroundings; thus, he could be satisfied anywhere. He had forgotten where the bathroom was, he needed to be led into the kitchen, and when it was time for bed, he no longer could find the bedroom. Alan only recognized his wife as someone who was kind to him, but Ellen knew that she could be kinder and gentler if she could sleep soundly, knowing that Alan was safe and cared for.

Ellen recognized that she needed to pay attention to herself, to be for herself and to care for herself. If she obeyed the Mishnah's challenge, she could be more sensitive to her husband's needs and could be a better partner for him. Alan was placed in a facility, and his wife now spends long, loving hours with him. She pays attention to his moods and makes sure that his medications are correct. Her presence ensures that staff members keep him clean and well nourished so that his skin is healthy, his muscles are exercised, and his care is as gentle and caring as possible. When she departs at night and goes to bed, Ellen sleeps soundly. How wonderful that, for Ellen, heeding her own needs benefited not only herself but her husband as well. "If I am for myself alone, what am I?"

The correct decisions for one patient with Alzheimer's are not necessarily the correct decisions for another patient with the same diagnosis. Like peeling an onion with layers coming off as the disease progresses, the social graces of patients tend to disappear and the underlying personality emerges. That is not always easy to deal with. The patient who had always been able to control or bury his instincts toward bigotry may begin using racial epithets. The patient who always was compliant with medical recommendations may begin to spit out pills. The patient who was demonstrative and loving may become resistant to being touched and angry if kissed. What appears at the core is not always pretty to see and can be embarrassing and distasteful. Families may shrink from awkward moments and often want to make institutional arrangements so that those moments don't happen again.

A patient with moderate dementia, Jack, lived with his daughter and son-in-law. His wife had died several years previously, and Jack was clueless about basic household tasks, such as cooking and doing laundry. That helplessness was exacerbated when he was diagnosed with dementia and when his daughter and son-in-law moved Jack into their home.

Jack went to a day program twice a week, and on other days he obediently trailed after his daughter as she went about her daily chores. One afternoon, his daughter Kathy needed some items from the local mall. After shopping, they waited in line to pay. Unfortunately, waiting was difficult for Jack; he had long ago forgotten the concept of "waiting one's turn." Instead, he quickly began swearing at the clerk. Jack told her that she was stupid and lazy, and he spoke in a loud enough voice for security to be called. Kathy was humiliated and tried to quiet her father, but of course, the more frantic she became, the more distressed he became and the situation escalated. Rather than calming down and explaining to security that Jack had dementia and was acting out of frustration, not intending to be hostile or aggressive, Kathy just wanted to get out of there. That was an understandable human emotion, but it wasn't helpful under the circumstances.

The inevitable outcome followed. Kathy felt she could never again risk taking Jack out in public, but she couldn't remain locked in her home with him, either. The decision was made to move him to a care facility. Jack didn't understand the situation, but once he was in his new surroundings, he knew that something had changed and he no longer knew where to find his daughter. Kathy was afraid to visit because she was afraid to overhear her father speak crudely to the aides.

Tragically, Kathy was for herself alone, not because she was a selfish or malevolent person, but because she was too personally overwrought to determine calmly what options might have been available to her. She also couldn't think through the possibility that others, such as the store clerk, might have their own relatives with dementia and might understand the havoc that dementia can wreak on personalities and internal, social controls.

Such a precipitous decision to move to placement happens frequently, and it rarely indicates that a caregiver is thoughtless or selfish. Sometimes it is absolutely appropriate and necessary. In Kathy's case, however, I am not certain that Jack needed placement as much as Kathy needed relief. She was frustrated. She was tired and exasperated and embarrassed with the unanticipated changes in her lifestyle that caring for Jack necessitated. More day care might have been too expensive, but possibly Kathy had other options, although she was too tired to seek them. Quite likely her synagogue or Jewish Family Service could have helped; the concept of a volunteer-based support system for dementia care in our communities has great merit. Perhaps Kathy needed Jack to occupy a respite bed periodically to give herself a chance to rest and regain perspective. And surely, a support group would have served her well.

Professionally, I hurt for couples like Kathy and her husband. They worked for years, longing for the time when their children would be through with college and they could relax and enjoy each other, only to discover that the end of their financial obligations to their children coincided with the beginning of their emotional and financial obligations to their parent with Alzheimer's disease. And, I hurt for spouses who similarly find that the end of their obligations to their children coincide with their partner being diagnosed with Alzheimer's disease.

"And, if not now, when?" When does my time come to enjoy life?" It is a natural cry of a heart. Sometimes, the next cry is, "How could you do this to me?" Cognitively, it makes no sense to blame the ill partner, but this is an emotional, gut-wrenching cry, and logic is irrelevant. Our feelings may have no basis in reality, but that doesn't make them less intense or less real.

The mishnah helps frame the questions. We need to ask: What are we if we think only of ourselves? Or, if we act out of desire simply to eliminate a problem—to let someone else deal with it—we need to ask if we are for ourselves, alone, and if so, what are we? Feelings are acceptable; acting hastily on those feelings can be hurtful when they have a direct, painful impact on someone else.

The examples I've offered are mostly from my professional practice as a geriatric care manager, but my own family has dealt with Alzheimer's disease. We're typical; few families are untouched by this epidemic. Cousin Arnold's illness tested my theories about families and stress, because providing care for him and keeping him content were very difficult. He could no longer comprehend his world, and he lost the ability to phrase his thoughts, and those losses were excruciating for him. He searched frantically for the nonexistent keys to make his world manageable again. And ultimately, he was institutionalized because we hoped that institutionalization would relieve him of the unrelenting pressure of searching. The family strongly supported Arnold's wife, Sue, in that decision, and it was the right thing to do. For Arnold, it worked.

14

He's Still My Father

MIKE COMINS

I know what others refuse to consider: my dad has dementia.

I know because when I returned to Los Angeles after a three-year stint in Wyoming, I used my parents' home as a base while I pursued my career as an itinerant rabbi and wilderness guide. We are working on my taxes. Dad's a CPA and a math whiz, but I am figuring out equations before him. I have almost never seen him cry, and now he tells me about an episode of *This American Life* and can't stop bawling. He never told a good story, but he could at least stay on track. Not now.

Nobody believes it because he clearly doesn't have a typical case of Alzheimer's. He forgets little. He never wanders. Rather, he is losing what was once his greatest strength: the ability to organize complicated scenarios, to frame the details in the context of the big picture. He can no longer put his thoughts in order sufficiently to answer the doctor's questions. He can't put together a shopping list.

My dad's dementia is as much physical as mental. His senses are slipping. He doesn't have Parkinson's, but he is quickly developing a tremor and losing his finer motor skills. Organizing his pills is now an emotionally draining ordeal. He can no longer dice an onion.

It's all very subtle. I wasn't sure until I read *The 36-Hour Day*[1] and learned the symptoms of dementia. When I bring it up with my mom, she is surprised and reacts harshly, even though my grandmother, my dad's mother, had Alzheimer's. "Everyone ages," she says. "He's seventy-six, after all! I wouldn't say dementia."

Dad visits the bathroom during the night, washes his hands, leaves the faucet on, and floods the dining room. The wooden floor is ruined.

People make mistakes. Any one of us might have done the same. By itself, I wouldn't have thought otherwise. But there is a pattern. His brain is changing, and so is he.

* * *

Then the unthinkable happens. My mother is diagnosed with stage-four liver cancer. We fuss over doctors and get the most aggressive treatment, hoping to give her a year instead of weeks. All attention is on her.

My dad is still driving, still working, still high functioning. But a truth of dementia is becoming evident as his situation worsens. The long, slow decline is anything but steady. It's more a matter of plateaus and valleys. Every so often, he seems to fall off a cliff into a more problematic state. He now sinks into periods of passive staring, a glassy look in his eyes.

But people can't see it. What would you look like if your wife of fifty years was about to die? Of course he's depressed and incapacitated. Why think dementia?

Besides, no one is paying much attention to him.

My own life is now officially on hold. I have proposed to my beloved Jody, but I am needed at home. We delay our wedding.

* * *

For the first time, Dad is conscious of the fact that he dreams. He gets up out of bed while dreaming and sleepwalks a bit, frightening himself when he wakes. He comes to me in a panic, asking me to help him figure it out. I tell him: dementia. He refuses that explanation.

On another night my parents are in bed and it hurts my mother to move, so she asks my father to pour her a glass of water from the pitcher on her dresser. Dad is in his semiconscious state, so instead of getting up and walking around the bed, he reaches over her body, knocks over the pitcher, and douses her. She is irate. My usually understanding mother is crying and pleading. Why can't he just not be lazy? All of the pain and unfairness of cancer is being directed at my father.

But he doesn't deserve it. He is ill, too. Only she doesn't believe it. And neither does he.

The chemo doesn't work. We spend Yom Kippur learning how to use my mother's new feeding tube.

* * *

I know that nothing would bring my mom greater joy than being at the wedding of her fifty-year-old bachelor son, but Jody and I don't want to start our married life living separately, and for now, I am taking care of my parents in their home.

It's good to be a rabbi. I know that the exchange of rings, originally an engagement ceremony, was held a year or more before the rest of the marriage ritual in ancient times. So we split our wedding ceremony in two. Jody and I gather with family and friends around my mom's bed the next day. My mother can no longer speak, but she smiles as the rabbi blesses us. We cry as we exchange rings and join our lives together.

My large extended family gathers in our house to congratulate us. In small groups, they visit my mom, who miraculously finds the strength to tell each of them, "I love you." I spend the evening arranging hospice care. It's unnecessary. She passes just before dawn.

We gather around the same bed, and my dad is in shock. His glassy eyes are wide open. He can't speak. He can't hear. He can't cry. He stares.

* * *

My mother spent all of two days on major painkillers and never slept a night in the hospital. She died in the arms of her daughter after witnessing her son's wedding, and she parted from her family with love. She died a heavenly death.

My dad's life becomes a living hell. He can't play cards with his grandsons or cook an omelet. His only defense is to believe nothing is wrong.

It is strange and ironic. I am now my dad's primary care manager. Both my siblings are closer to him, but one lives in another city, and the other has a business and kids. So it's me.

A lot of firstborn children rebel against their parents, but I was extreme. My dad was a CPA; I took my last math class in tenth grade and turned to writing and the humanities. Dad had little interest in religion; I became a rabbi. He was quiet; I was a public speaker and youth group president. He hated team sports; I played on the high school football team.

In my child's mind, I rebelled because I couldn't stomach that my father was the class nerd, the scrawniest guy on the block, the butt of too many jokes. It didn't bother him much. He was smarter than most everyone else, married the prettiest girl, and did very well in business. He hiked and jogged. But I was a child who wanted my father to be a hero.

* * *

The neurologist holds the report from the brain scan. My dad's shrinking brain is consistent with moderate to severe Alzheimer's. "I don't believe it," Dad says. The doctor agrees. He's still getting twenty-six out of thirty on the memory test. So how does the scan correspond with reality?

"Oh, you really do have dementia," the doctor tells my dad. "It's just not that bad, yet."

So he continues to fool almost everybody. He recognizes people. He remembers. He converses. He can think sophisticated thoughts. He goes to his office every day, where his partners graciously indulge him. You could easily think that he's just slowed down. I'd say that too if I didn't see him at home, where he struggles to sort out his pills from his vitamins and can't follow the plot of a movie.

* * *

I think of us, and I think of Isaac and Esau. The least heroic of the biblical Patriarchs, Isaac loves his older son, Esau, the athlete, the hunter who prefers solitude in the wilderness to the gossip at home. As a blind old man, he gets duped by his wife, Rebecca, and Jacob, his younger son.

Or does he?

Isaac wants to bless his children, we are told, because he is old and fading. He must formally pass the mantle of leadership before he dies. While Esau is hunting for the fresh game that Isaac has requested, Jacob tries to fool him. He masquerades as his hairy brother by wearing an animal hide. But Isaac recognizes Jacob's voice. Would he really have been deceived by a goat's skin? Or did he have his own agenda? Perhaps Isaac gave each son exactly what he wanted to give them.

I like to think so. Isaac, like my dad, was coping as best he could. And appearances can be deceiving. When Jacob returns from his sojourn with Laban twenty years later, Isaac is still alive.

* * *

I tell my dad that the situation is untenable. Jody and I have scheduled our wedding ceremony, part two, and I need to move out. Dad can't cook for himself. He has virtually no social life. Surely he should be in a place where his meals are prepared and around people he can befriend.

But the obvious alternative, an assisted-living facility, is unspeakable. His friends are fond of saying they'd rather die than move into one. You only go there if your life is over. I'd like to rake them over the coals.

For a while Dad's condition improves as the trauma of my mother's death recedes. No more blank stares or spacing out at the dinner table. But over time, his symptoms worsen. He can no longer do much at work. He is agitated in a crowd. He can't play in the family Scrabble games or tell a story in conversation. He seems to be okay, but it's like he took a stupid pill.

The overwhelming impulse is to be angry with him. Clearly his memory is okay; we can't help thinking that if he wanted to enough, if he would just try a little harder, he could be the man we all know.

Now that I've studied the disease, my frustration rarely makes me angry. But his friends, relatives, and acquaintances don't know much about dementia, and they haven't been around him enough to see that he has it. They get annoyed. They get angry. He puts them in the awkward position of having to patronize an old friend whose mind had once commanded so much respect. Mostly, they're shocked and sad, and they don't want to admit it. So they blame him. Why can't he fix it? They blame me. Why can't I fix him? Obviously, I'm not paying enough attention to him or taking him to the right doctors. I can't blame them. I thought the same way before I learned about the disease. But I can't stop thinking that we should be able to fix this, as well. And since I know better, I get mad at myself.

* * *

Some days Dad agrees with everything I say and admits that he has dementia. And then there are the other days. Driving him home from a doctor's appointment, I pull into an intersection too quickly. I slam on the brakes to avoid the cross traffic. "See," he says, "you're a worse driver than I am." At that moment, it's hard to argue the point.

The months go by. My brother and sister have stepped up. We all take care of Dad. But that allows him to remain in denial. We can't make him plan for a disease that he can't admit he has. We could force him to move into a home, but if we take away his ability to decide where he'll live, what will we have done to his person, to his selfhood, to his humanity? Will we still have a "father"; will I still be his "son"?

I hear an interview with an Alzheimer's patient on the radio. The woman can't remember her son's name. She rationalizes that she *chooses* not to use it. "I've always called you 'son.'" So it goes. How else does a person hold on to her self-esteem and not give in to the disease?

"See, I set before you this day life and prosperity, death and adversity. . . . Choose life," states Deuteronomy (30:15, 30:19). That he won't leave his home is an act of enormous stupidity immersed in outrageous denial, and yet, it is his most powerful way of "choosing life." He is holding on to the person that he wants to be, the healthy, happy face he still sees in the mirror. He won't throw in the towel.

I now have an entirely new understanding of "Honor your father and your mother" (Exodus 20:12). There is no clear, right way, and every choice carries life-threatening risks. I must restrain myself and live with the knowledge that whatever the choices that are made, he is in either psychological or physical danger, or both. To honor my father is to accept this unending state of uncertainty and to live with fear.

* * *

Despite his objections, I force him to attend a support group at the Alzheimer's Association, hoping he will see the light and move into an assisted-living facility.

He doesn't want to be there, and neither do I. Each participant is there with a spouse, except for my dad. He has a son, and his son will never care for him like a spouse.

My heart goes out to these spouses. They feel so much responsibility. They can't delegate care to hired hands or send their loved ones to an assisted-living facility. They hold on, even when their demented spouse no longer knows who they are.

I feel good for my mother. I see how much suffering her untimely death has spared her. And unlike these spouses, I never suffer the indignity of my dad not recognizing me. No, it is my dad who bears the greatest suffering.

For most Alzheimer's victims, anger and anxiety eventually give way to a lost-in-space bliss that is terribly disturbing to a loved one, but not so painful to the demented one. My dad's memory, however, is still good. He is fully aware. And he can't keep his dignity while admitting what he knows every day, every hour, every minute. Something has gone terribly wrong.

There is no understanding dementia in an objective way. My father just knows his life is being taken from him and he can't stop it. He doesn't understand how it happened, or why it happened to him. It's all an unbelievable nightmare, and he is aware of it every moment. It is not my mother, nor I or my siblings, nor his friends who bear this dark, relentless, unforgiving burden. Unlike the Alzheimer's patient who lives in his own world, Dad suffers beyond imagination.

The result is predictable. Depression becomes as difficult as the dementia. Over the next few years, we try three different antidepressant medications. They work wonders with other members of the support group. Dad can't tolerate any of them.

* * *

I feel like I did years ago when I served in the Israeli army, doing reserve duty. I guarded Palestinian prisoners. It caused me a lot of mental anguish, but I just repressed it. Despite all the kvetching that Israelis revel in, it's not okay to complain about reserve duty. There's an unwritten rule: everyone goes through this; the country will fall apart if we can't do our jobs in the reserves; do your duty; don't whine.

It seems that everyone and his brother has a loved one with dementia. Who am I to complain? Look at other people. At least my dad still knows who I am. I'm lucky.

* * *

A year after my mother's death, the wedding approaches and I move out. I know the suffering it causes my dad. And I know the risk. But he'll never agree to move to an assisted-living facility until his children stop enabling him to pretend that he's self-sufficient.

We fear every drive he takes to buy a hamburger, and we listen to him explain how much he likes the hot dogs that he makes at home. Before, I'd never seen him boil a hot dog, even once.

When he finally agrees to leave, he accuses me of forcing him. I take him to visit the facility closest to me, the best in terms of staffing and level of care. But he is still his own man, and that's the point he wants to get across. He chooses a place in the opposite direction, farther from the few friends who would visit him and farther from me, the one who takes care of him the most. It is totally irrational to an outside observer and totally irrational to me. Three years later, it still angers me.

I don't want to admit that what appeared to me to be the wrong decision was in fact the right decision for him or that I admire him for it. In his mind, not giving in to the disease means not giving in to my arguments for a place with an Alzheimer's program and increased medical care, for that would mean admitting he's really sick and getting worse. How can I blame him? He's fighting for his life. I would have done the same. But it doesn't change the fact. The person most invested in his care will visit him half as much.

* * *

I look at my favorite picture of the family. We are backpacking. Two thirty-something parents with three kids, ages six to twelve, traversing the Sierra Nevada mountains. My dad, the butt of all the jokes, is the Moses taking his family into the unforgiving wild, where hospitals are far away. If you listened to him talk later in life, you'd never have thought that he would take us into the backcountry. In general, he is a fearful man. But we, his family, knew the warrior in him.

We seem so opposite, my dad and I, especially to me. But today I know that we are not so different. He loved the life I led. He supported the adventures of his high school football league MVP, Israeli soldier, and desert guide son. He was a CPA, and yet he never complained (to me anyway) about my disregard for financial security.

I always thought he didn't understand me, but now I think he was like Isaac.

Why did Isaac, the most passive of the Patriarchs, love the brash, impulsive man of the desert, his son, Esau? The Jewish mystical text the *Zohar* explains, "Everyone loves his own kind—the one who is similar to himself."[2]

On the surface, it seems that passive Isaac is more like Jacob, who prefers life in the tents to the challenges of the wilderness, who spends his life running from Esau and Laban. But just like my dad, there's more to the story. The only patriarch who never left the Land of Israel, Isaac held his own in the face of dangerous threats from powerful neighbors. The fields he sowed reaped a hundredfold harvest. He led with a quiet courage and tenacious resolve. He wasn't passive at all.

If you saw my dad backpacking, you knew what his clients knew. He was no pushover. How easy for me, blessed with athletic skill, to take on a physical challenge. Not so my Dad; but hiking was his love, and he literally led his family through the wilderness.

I grew up thinking that my life was a rebellion against his. On many levels, it is. But not where it counts. He blessed me with the gifts that led to my life as an outdoor educator. I followed in his footsteps. Just as Esau was in his father Isaac's heart, I am in my dad's.

And he is in mine.

* * *

In his famous compilation of Jewish law, the *Mishneh Torah*, Maimonides, the twelfth-century rabbi, philosopher, and physician, writes, "There is also a *sefer Torah shebalah*, a Torah scroll in which one letter after another becomes faded and disappears, until there is nothing left. But even though that Torah scroll can no longer be used for reading in the synagogue, it must be treated with dignity, and buried with respect."[3]

My dad is now in the dementia ward at the assisted-living facility near me. He can no longer hold a conversation or stand up by himself, and he often needs to be fed. We, his children, don't know how better to respect him. But he hates it—like a Torah scroll, I imagine, that can't fulfill its essential task: to be read.

The one physical enjoyment left, food, is subpar. He's surrounded by demented people, many of whom have completely lost their minds; some yell and scream. But whenever I enter the room his eyes light up and he says, "Mike!" and he laughs the quiet chuckle of a laugh he has laughed all his life. He won't sit still, and though he's often in his own world now, he spends most every waking moment on his walker, determined to get to a destination he cannot name and will never reach.

Maybe he's fulfilling his essential task. He's moving. He's willing himself forward. He's not giving in.

He's hiking.

I'm still trying to keep up.

15

⁓❦⁓

The Uncertain Path:
Emerging Issues for the Caregiver

RICHARD F. ADDRESS

I

"Who are you?"

Better to ask, I think, "*Where* are you?"

It is a well-staffed, caring nursing home that specializes in dementia patients. My mother has been a resident for close to a year. My, how time flies. I remember the call from her assisted-living facility. It came while I was in the middle of teaching a class at Hebrew Union College. The message was clear: something has happened, and your mother is being transported to a local hospital. The diagnosis was "changed mental status," and during that week in the hospital, my mother transitioned into a new state of being that, tragically, defines all too many. For months we negotiated treatment issues, wound our way through the labyrinth of Medicaid eligibility, and endured two additional emergency trips to the hospital; each brought with it an aftermath of further reduced cognition and strength. There are good days and bad days, visits where we can actually engage in some sort of conversation. And there are visits when we sit in silent vigil, staring at this once vital, independent businesswoman who is now a frail, bedridden fragile shadow of what once was. "Where are you, Mom? It's me, your son!"

Perhaps it is the stare that we see when we visit. It is glassy-eyed and filled with a sadness that defies description. It is almost as if there is a sense that, behind that stare, there is some sort of understanding that this is not right, that no one is meant to "live" like this. Yet, there is animation and emotion, especially when her great-granddaughter comes to visit Bubbe. This little girl sits on my mother's bed and leans close, singing a song learned that week in preschool. There is a smile on my mother's face. The cycle of life? Who can say anything other than there is still a soul there, locked in some prison of dementia, but still there, somewhere.

I am not alone. In my work in developing the Reform Movement's Sacred Aging project, I have met hundreds of people who shared this journey. They reported on the challenges of being a caregiver, of juggling work and family and of trying to manage the medical system. They found themselves subject to a range of emotions, sometimes all at the same time, and they sought comfort and support whenever and wherever possible. One young woman who was beginning this new life stage wrote:

> Being a caregiver is never easy. We are constantly being asked to give of ourselves, with little time to take a breath and sort out our own emotions. We are overrun with the big and the little, never knowing which should take precedence. We feel silly and dramatic when worrying about how the health and well-being of another affect us, yet we know that it does change our lives. Being a caregiver to a parent only raises the ante on all these emotions and questions.[1]

Caregiving elicits a wealth of stories. I encountered what I've found to be a typical example after finishing a workshop on how congregations could respond to issues of dementia and Alzheimer's. Myron, a man in his seventies, approached me and asked if we could just sit and talk for a while. He told me his story and, after some prodding, agreed to have it shared. He spoke of his wife and of the moment when he watched her cradle a doll while at the same time not recognizing her youngest daughter's voice when she called on the phone. He shared his story of having to face the rapid decline in his wife's condition. No two journeys are the same, and we realize that while there may be similarities in cases, no two family stories are the same. Myron continued to weave a story of frustration and confusion as he reflected on the stages he went through, from initial denial to anger and beyond:

> All the years of work and planning for retirement—our trips, our sharing getting old together, our enjoyment of our children and grandchildren—all going up in smoke. As my wife is gradually but inexorably disappearing, despair and sadness have supplanted anger. More recently I have been able to move to a state of hope and regain some clarity around the future. I now hope I can provide an environment that will be safe for my wife, while still recognizing the need for my life to continue. Although I refer to these emotional stages as sequential, I often move back and forth among the various stages. Everyone I have spoken to has made the same two suggestions: surround yourself with a support network and look after yourself. Both are easier said than done.

The revolution in longevity that now embraces us has given us untold possibilities for personal growth and social transformation. It also has raised significant ethical questions as to what longevity can mean. As the baby-boom generation enters its own process of aging, and with the blessings of medical technology and a greater awareness of health all around us, boomers can look forward to, God willing, a life expectancy well into one's eighties or nineties or more. With that blessing also comes the curse of more instances of Alzheimer's and dementia. As a society, we are nowhere near ready to assume these challenges. Implicit in these challenges are issues of caregiving: not only care for people who are afflicted with these conditions, but also caring for the caregivers. Alzheimer's and related conditions can last for years, perhaps decades, and the management of these situations can overwhelm a person and a family, especially as the caregivers themselves age. Yet, these scenarios also can provide opportunities for the creation of new types of support programs and even rituals and prayers that speak to the challenges inherent in coping with these new realities.

There is no shortage of resources that speak to the psycho-spiritual challenges of being a caregiver. There is a shortage, though, of resources that speak to the spiritual aspects of how this life stage of caregiver can be a possible source of creative ritual or programming. Thankfully, increasing numbers of social service organizations and religious institutions are developing support programs for families and individuals who are dealing with dementia and/or Alzheimer's disease. These groups provide needed human contact and opportunities for sharing of stories, challenges, and practical information. However, the question that is slowly surfacing is how a religious institution can or should try to respond to these family issues.

A few scenarios come to mind. Right now there are untold numbers of individuals, our loved ones, who reside at facilities that care for people with dementia or Alzheimer's. They may be in their fifties or in their nineties. One thing is certain, however: they will not be returning to their previous life, and as time evolves, they slowly fade away on what seems to some to be a long, slow dance to death. On the one hand, they are alive and with us, and on another, they have left us. I began to understand this limbo several months after my mother was placed into her nursing home. I was speaking to a therapist who has helped guide my journey, and I remarked that it had occurred to me that I had begun the process of mourning my mother's death when she was placed in the nursing home. It hit me that although she was still alive and with us, she was slipping away, and we all knew what the end would be. It was as if my soul had begun the process of mourning, even though no actual death was in the immediate future. It felt strange and somewhat discomforting. I was searching for some term or label to put on this feeling. A fellow traveler on this road wrote of his similar experience and found a term that described this state. He referred to it as "ambiguous loss." He explained:

> Although all losses are touched with ambiguity, those who suffer ambiguous loss, losses without finality or resolution, bear a particular and challenging burden. One form of ambiguous loss involves physical presence and psychological absence. Such ambiguous loss can occur in dementia which takes a loved one's mind

and memory away. In this type of ambiguous loss, the person you care about is psychologically absent—that is emotionally and cognitively missing. As there is no end to ambiguous loss, it freezes the grief process and prevents closure; it tends to paralyze functioning. Tensions build up as experiencing ambiguous loss can cause conflicting thoughts and feelings. We may dread the death of a loved one who is hopelessly ill while at the same time longing for closure and an end to waiting. Such feelings inevitably cause guilt. As family members of patients with dementia, we can be both angry and sad; angry at the demands of care-giving, while at the same time sad because we are losing a loved one.

Futhermore, there are no community-sanctioned farewell rituals such as funerals or shivas to comfort family members experiencing the loss of their loved one to dementia. Of all losses experienced in personal relationships, ambiguous loss remains the most devastating because it remains unclear and indeterminate.[2]

The ever-increasing number of those having to care for people with dementia or Alzheimer's demands that religious institutions address the issues of the caregiver's psycho-spiritual support. One still-powerful way to open this conversation is to use the "power of the pulpit." Congregations have begun to create Shabbat services that honor caregivers. Rabbis have begun to preach on what it is like to walk through this wilderness and, as so many do, feel so alone. Raising this issue also allows for sharing personal thoughts.

We observe our loved ones in this strange, new existence and we wonder what may be the limits of treatment, how aggressive or passive may we be in treating infections or complications that may emerge from their evolving frailty. This, of course, is another reason why it is incumbent on everyone to have a medical advance directive as well as a health care proxy power of attorney. Our wishes need to be known and made clear to family, clergy, and physicians, and those wishes and these documents *must* be reexamined and updated on a regular basis. This has become, thanks to the miracles of medical technology, a modern mitzvah.

But what of the spiritual basis for this decision making? Judaism is somewhat clear regarding end-of-life scenarios. The life stage called *goseis* (a moribund person whose death is near at hand, i.e., a person in late-stage hospice care) does not apply to someone with dementia or Alzheimer's, who may not be anywhere near imminent death. Are we commanded to do everything in our power to be aggressive in treating such a person? And, do our answers depend on the case before us? Is it different for an Alzheimer's patient of age fifty-five, who may be expected to live years, if not decades, than for a woman in her nineties? The bioethics literature of Judaism is filled with guidance regarding end-of-life situations. The *goseis* category, which focuses on a death that is imminent, has been supplemented by the examination of another legal term: *terefah*. This is a concept concerning someone who may be living with a terminal illness but who, thanks to medical technology, is functioning and living life. Their death also is nowhere near imminent. Elliot Dorff contrasts this term with that of a person being *goseis* by noting that "the appropriate Jewish legal category to describe people who have incurable diseases but who may live for months, or even years is, instead, *terefah* (an imperiled life), that is, a person having been diagnosed as having a terminal illness."[3]

However, my sense is that the mood of Jewish biomedical thought, even concerning *terefah*, focuses more on the seriously ill person. Is someone living with dementia or Alzheimer's in the category of *terefah*? Jewish tradition allows for nonaggressive treatment of certain conditions in cases of *terefah* and *goseis*. Does the same concept hold for the Alzheimer's patient of age sixty-five who is living in a care facility? Or do we need to develop another definition from Jewish tradition that best describes these situations? I also would argue against the use of the traditional term of *shoteh* (from Babylonian Talmud, *Chagigah* 3b), which describes one who is mentally incompetent. The context of the Talmudic discussion refers to a person's ability or inability to be called as a witness at a court (*beit din*). Was Myron's wife "mentally incompetent"? Is there a difference between the person dealing with mental illness and the person with dementia or Alzheimer's? In one sense—that they are cognitively failing—yes, they could both be considered *shoteh*. Yet, does that adequately and fairly describe Myron's wife, my mother, or the people with dementia we all may know? It is time for our community, in light of the revolution in longevity and the blessings of medical technology, to seek a new Jewish legal term that with love and care can better describe this elongated state of life that so many of our loved ones now endure and that so many of us may come to experience.

The tradition gives us an insight into one possibility. One of the classic terms used to describe aspects of mental illness is the term *teiruf hadaat*, which can be understood as a "tearing away of knowledge." That is what happens in cases of dementia or Alzheimer's. One's knowledge of the world and of the self is torn away. Perhaps this Talmudic term can be applied to these cases. There is a Modern Hebrew term for dementia, *shit'yon*, derived from the above-mentioned *shoteh*, yet less severe, and which seems to reflect a generic, more clinical definition. One can make the case, given our current and evolving demographics, that we can see in *teiruf hadaat* a category of person who has entered this stage of the long good-bye, a life stage that will require us to examine modes of care as well as become educated and active in the spiritual and legal guidelines that are desired to care for a loved one.

II

The Jewish legal status of a loved one suffering from Alzheimer's or dementia and the difficulties faced by his or her caregivers is a challenge not only for legal scholars and bioethicists, but for every person engaged in Jewish communal life. In response to this challenge, the Union for Reform Judaism's Department of Jewish Family Concerns initiated the Sacred Aging project to create resources for congregations on the emerging revolution in longevity now under way within our community. Among the unexpected consequences of the Sacred Aging project were discussions that focused on the need to look at new Jewish rituals that spoke to the issues dealt with by caregivers.

One of the more controversial issues centered around the healthy, well spouse finding someone to share moments of emotional, spiritual, and physical intimacy. We learned of many cases involving a man or woman whose spouse had been confined to a facility for a very long time. Children were grown and living their own lives. The caregiver spouse always was attentive and involved in the caring of the spouse who was ill. Yet, as time passed, these individuals reported that their own sense of aloneness and isolation began to take a profound toll. For some, the development of a new intimate relationship provided a healing balm. Was this adultery? Were they guilty of some grave sin, or were they seeking a psycho-spiritual haven to help them through their journey? This scenario is no longer an isolated circumstance. I suggest that it is more prevalent than we may wish to admit, and given the current demographics and trends within our community and, as noted, the expected rise in cases of Alzheimer's and dementia as baby boomers age and live longer, this scenario will become more common. It is important, then, for us to develop a new understanding of this elongated stage of illness that will allow for the Jewish community to recognize this new, very real relationship in a meaningful and, hopefully, nonjudgmental manner. Also, it is important for our community to similarly consider ways in which to be sensitive to the spouses who do choose to travel this new road. It may be time, in light of the advances in technology and the reality of the new demographics, to consider the creation, *in certain contexts*, of a redefinition of adultery.

One can only imagine the emotional stresses and strains that are involved in such situations. I believe that the time has come for congregations to become involved in this issue. Just as we develop programming to assist in preparing advance medical directives, I suggest that the time is at hand to create a document that allows couples to discuss their actions and desires in situations where one may be institutionalized with Alzheimer's or dementia, which may include permission for the healthy spouse to develop new intimate relationships even while the demented spouse remains alive. Will this be for everyone? No. Could it be helpful to many? Perhaps. I believe so, if for no other reason than it will allow the discussion to take place. Has such a document ever been developed? Yes. It was called "An Open Letter to My Spouse," and it asked couples to take the time to seriously consider the emotional needs that may arise in moments of extreme crises. The "Open Letter" makes a fundamental assumption that the couple will love and care for each other yet understand that conditions may arise, totally unforeseen, that may alter the relationship. A major part of the document speaks to our issue and states:

> As medical science, nutrition and exercise, and a host of other factors conspire successfully to allow the average American to live longer, the chances get better and better that I will be "alive" in body, but possibly significantly compromised mentally and/or physically. Loving me as you do, I know that you will care for me to the best of your ability. But, if I am compromised, and unable to maybe even recognize you or remember that we are married, you will be faced with a double burden: additional stress of caring for me in my sad state, and the absence of my emotional, physical, and intellectual support. I hope that this does not happen, but if it does, I want you to know that I will want you to do the best you can to be supported by a loving companion. Please find someone you like who will be available to provide the emotional, intellectual, and physical support and companionship that I cannot provide to you.[4]

The idea of examining the possible creation of new approaches to how we view relationships in extraordinary situations has had some discussion within the organized Jewish world. An article by Rabbi J. David Bleich, in an Orthodox Jewish journal, considered a category of relationship referred to as *derech kiddushin* (in the manner of marriage), which could be used as a foundation for new definitions of relationships that emerge in catastrophic circumstances.[5] Rabbi Daniel Schiff, writing in a compendium of Reform articles on marriage, opened the door for this discussion in looking at what he called "circumstantial adultery" that emerges in cases of serious physical or mental impairment of a spouse. "If the spouse of the comatose patient finds a committed partner with whom a sexual relationship is shared, adultery will be the result, though it is an adultery that arguably might warrant a moral response different from that given to other categories."[6]

As a result of these articles and in direct response to numerous discussions in workshops regarding new rituals for aging baby boomers, a template document has been developed. This document grew out of the Union for Reform Judaism's Sacred Aging project and is an attempt to provide a basis for conversation and discussion within congregations. It examines a reinterpretation of the traditional concept of the *agunah*, the spouse who is left in a limbo state as a result of a spouse who is missing. (This category of limbo, or *agunah*, more commonly was experienced in earlier times, especially when a husband was presumed but not confirmed to have died while away on a voyage, a journey, or in battle, thus rendering the surviving wife as abandoned and trapped, unable to legally remarry until or unless the spouse was confirmed as deceased.) This new document considers the possibility that a spouse who is institutionalized with Alzheimer's and/or dementia has, in a very real way, gone missing and that his or her essence is no longer there; he or she has metaphorically abandoned the living spouse as a virtual *agunah*.[7]

The purpose of developing such a document is not merely to allow people to do what they want when they want; rather, it is to hope that congregations will see in this an issue that is impacting increasing numbers in our community. Just the fact that the conversation about the role of the caregiving spouse is brought forward may provide comfort and support. Also, this may encourage communities to actually stimulate open and honest conversation with people, while they are both healthy, so that the issue can be explored and feelings expressed. At the very least, we can bring forward the conversation regarding when a person becomes *teiruf hadaat* and what actions by the caregiving spouse or partner may be more generally accepted, given the severity of the circumstances.

There is no doubt that this can be viewed as challenging and to some, controversial; to others, it is a matter of personal privacy. This is not for everyone! There will be those in our community who will see these discussions as totally out of the purview of Jewish life. Yet the actions resulting from individuals and families who are now living and experiencing these caregiving realities cannot be ignored. They are our congregants, our friends and family, and they are, or in many cases will be, us. To ignore their struggles and challenges may be to deprive them of the care and support that a living and dynamic faith can offer.

16

The Not-Person

DOUGLAS J. KOHN

Losing anything is upsetting—losing your keys, forgetting a phone number, misplacing an umbrella. It is especially upsetting because you know that the desired object is not far away. And, if losing an object or a single piece of information is upsetting, then losing a family member or a dear one is surely the most disquieting of all losses. Even more upsetting is losing that dear one while he or she is present and still very much alive and functioning; he or she is failing and, like the keys or the umbrella, is not far away. Such is the insidious nature of Alzheimer's disease: it steals the inner being of one's father or mother, spouse or sibling or grandparent, right from under one's nose—day by day, memory by memory, ability by ability. We lose them as they sit before us. And, yet, as that person—or that person's mind and memory—erodes and atrophies, we may ask, what becomes of his or her *person*? Where does the *person* go, the one whom we once knew and who once knew us? The shell is still present, the physical vessel of his or her being, the living, functioning body; but surely the *person* is eroded, lost, elsewhere.

How does Judaism help us to understand where the *person* has gone, while leaving behind the empty—or emptying—shell? The Mishnah, our second-century code of Jewish law, offers a prescription regarding a human person: *B'makom she-ein anashim, hishtadeil lih'yot ish*, "In a place where there is no humanity, strive to be a human being" (*Pirkei Avot* 2:5). Yet, when the human being can no longer strive, and even recedes before the onslaught of Alzheimer's disease, and little if any humanity remains, what can we understand of that person?

Such was the case of David Kohn, my grandfather, and of Jack Bloom, my father-in-law (each of blessed memory). In many ways, Grandpa and Jack were very similar persons. Both were working men—Grandpa in welding and hardware in New Jersey, and Jack a produce broker in Philadelphia—and though neither had more than a high school education, each had a sharp, analytical mind, was able with numbers, and had an abiding sense of justice. As well, each basically was a gentle and reserved man. And, both developed Alzheimer's disease at about the same time: Grandpa's diagnosis came a number of years after he retired to Florida, and Jack's came rather prematurely as he was concluding his working career, and he was forced to sell his business and begin a new and unsettling chapter of life.

As they nearly simultaneously descended into Alzheimer's dementia, circumstances allowed that I spent far more time with my father-in-law than with my grandfather. In order that my wife and our young family could be closer to her parents and to participate, moderately, in Jack's care, I left my then rabbinic post for a new congregational position that was nearer her family. Admittedly, I saw Grandpa much too infrequently, and thus I was shocked by the dramatic losses—his shrinkage into but a distant shell. I did, however, experience Jack's steady and uneasy decline, his seven-year descent into a distant, angry, clumsy husk of his former self. As a young husband and rabbi, I was deeply stricken by the loss of each of their personhoods. What happened to the playful grandfather who had always awakened early to read the paper and then walk to the grocer, get milk, and cook pancakes for his still slumbering grandchildren? To where disappeared that grandfather's once smiling *punim* behind that scruffy mustache, as he sat unresponsive in a nondescript lounge in the "old-age home" in Fort Lauderdale, unable to recognize or discourse with his grandson? And, what of the brilliant produce broker who once could tally a towering column of figures with only a sharpened pencil and a scrap of paper and who had lovingly worried over the well-being of every distant family member? Where was that Jack, who now lumbered about the house with a shuffling zombie's gait, periodic unprovoked agitation, and an automaton's empty stare? Yes, what of my father-in-law, who only years earlier had been thoughtful, witty, playful, and a perfect gentleman, but who now blurted non sequiturs and spurted obscenities from his unrepressed mouth, which evidently no longer was managed by his previously superb self-control?

Where were the wonderful persons whom I had adored, respected, and loved? Surely, their bodies were there, but their beings, their persons, had been eviscerated. When Alzheimer's disease robs a soul of its mind and memory, what can we understand of that person?

Moses Maimonides (called the Rambam), the twelfth-century Spanish philosopher, Talmud commentator, and physician, included in his commentary on the Mishnah a psycho-spiritual document titled *Sh'monah P'rakim*, which also is called *A Treatise on the Soul*. In it, Maimonides argued that a soul distinguishes what is alive from that which is not alive, that the soul (*nefesh*, in Hebrew) was the body in operation, and that the *nefesh*, the core of a person, required rational skills and knowledge. He wrote, citing a verse from the Book of Proverbs, "'Also, the soul without knowledge is not good' [Prov. 19:2] . . . The verse teaches that it would not be proper for a soul [*nefesh*] to remain without knowledge and thus not to fulfill its form."[1] To Rambam, a person was the operations of his soul, and those operations were based primarily in reason and intellect. Thus, we understand the corollary, that when a soul has lost the ability to reason or the capacity to harness its intellect, it could cease to be an operating soul.

Although we would admit that Rambam practiced a relatively primitive form of medicine, his explanation of the soul as the seat of a human person's mind offers a spiritual understanding of the losses that come with Alzheimer's disease, especially the losses of memory and cognitive ability. Rambam taught that the soul is grounded in both knowledge and reasoning, and without either, the person sinks into something lesser. As I observed both my grandfather and my father-in-law suffer the depravations of Alzheimer's disease, I saw them relinquish their grip on reason and knowledge, and their souls therefore become something lesser than human souls.

Early in his Alzheimer's descent, Jack was still talkative and gentlemanly, and once he and my mother-in-law, Meye, came to town for a visit. Although Jack was still rather high functioning, traveling was disorienting and taxing. Thus, when I was going out to play golf with a congregant, Meye suggested that I take Jack along, as he once had been a prolific golfer, and the experience could be pleasant. I was concerned but agreeable, so when Jack also agreed and rode along in my golf cart, offering to me and my buddy some clear, cogent advice on the golf grip, and lining up and hitting the ball, I was thoroughly surprised. Out on the golf course, Jack's captive soul was temporarily liberated, and he was unexpectedly buoyant, spirited, and self-assured. Meye could hardly believe it when I reported back that afternoon! However, it was heartrending. It was a teasing and fleeting glimpse backward through the looking glass at a soul that was momentarily reawakened and that would soon thereafter retreat back to its imposing darkness.

Yet, for me, the experience on the golf course was evidence of the teachings of both the Mishnah and Rambam. Inside my father-in-law's emptying mind and soul, like a balloon losing its precious air pressure, this was a brief moment of striving. "In a place where there is no humanity, *hishtadeil lih'yot ish*—strive to be a human being." I was treated to my father-in-law striving and retrieving a brief measure of his leaking humanity, and it warmed and stirred me, and remains a prized memory, even years later, after his death in 1995. Furthermore, somehow overcoming the arresting plaque and shrinking recesses of his then-suffering brain, Jack's golf memories remained strong and surprisingly accessible and were triggered that day. Likely he hadn't been on a golf course for many years, yet when he returned to that place on which he had spent so many happy and stimulating—or frustrating—hours, a part of his mind reawakened. Rambam would explain that this was Jack's soul in form and operation, with years of accumulated golf knowledge and wisdom. I was treated to a rare and treasured sighting of this man's operating soul—treasured even when he yelled, "Fore!" and laughed after one of my errant shots—which soon would be thoroughly lost.

But my father-in-law clearly was waning. He would have fewer and fewer moments of striving to be a human being, of his soul operating to form. Meye was determined to keep him at home, and she gallantly resisted placing Jack in a care facility, even if it meant that she would be an exhausted caregiver. At times, helpers and respite workers would come to the house, but primarily, Meye was the bather, feeder, entertainer, and worrier, as more than once Jack wandered off and was found by the police, roving lost in the neighborhood. Meye became active with the local chapter of the Alzheimer's Association and even would be honored as their Volunteer of the Year. Yet, Jack was waning and soon would be constrained to a special chair. The former produce broker, who once claimed Philadelphia's finest restaurateurs among his clients, was now fed baby food.

What of his person?

Late in the Book of Deuteronomy, when Moses is preparing to die, he offers a final farewell to the people he has shepherded through the desert for forty years. Although he was 120 years old, the Torah recounts that he had not suffered physical or mental failures in his old age. Knowing that he was about to die, Moses implores his wandering Jews to remember the devotion of God and offers this poetic charge: "Remember the days of old, / Consider the years of ages past; / Ask your parent, who will inform you, / Your elders, who will tell you" (Deuteronomy 32:7). Moses is fearful that the Jews will soon forget his teachings and the miraculous, redemptive wonders wrought on their behalf by God, so he urges them to seek their elders, who will serve as their institutional memory. Clearly, if Moses at 120 years of age could recall and narrate all the events of the previous four decades, then surely he might assume, the other elders could do likewise. Yet, Moses was unique. Although there is no textual record of Alzheimer's disease among Moses's most aged Israelites, we can imagine that there must have been many whose minds and memories were fading with illness, brain plaque, neurofibrillary tangles, and shrinkage, whose souls were no longer operating to form, and who could not serve as institutional or even family memory. Thus, Moses's poetic verse is also a poignant verse: "Ask your parent, who will inform you, / Your elders, who will tell you."

What of the person? Ultimately, when the parent can no longer inform you or the elder no longer tell you, when cognitive and functional impairment becomes pronounced and irreversible, and memory and thinking skills are destroyed and even the simplest tasks are unable to be undertaken, the person ceases to be the person he or she was. We may resist acknowledging it, even as we very much realize and recognize it. There are very clear behavioral and cognitive symptoms and changes, but the shell of the person is still largely intact, so we are hesitant to despair. And, because there may be moments of wonderful clarity and even beauty, like the afternoon on the golf course with Jack, we still cling to hope and optimism with tenacity. Yet, the *nefesh*, the soul of the person, the *ish* to whom one strives to be in one's fullest moments, is waning and not functioning to form.

It was so very difficult to observe or engage my father-in-law while he was restrained in the special chair. It was a large, cushioned medical chair in uninspiring teal faux-leather vinyl, with a high back and neck cushions to protect against Jack accidentally falling backwards or sideways. As well, the chair had a tray that could be clipped to its arms, on which food could be placed. Also, frequently found on Jack's tray would be any number of playing cards, randomly lying faceup or facedown. Jack no longer played cards or even knew what the cards signified, but he could occupy himself for periods by moving the cards from side to side or from pile to pile. It usually required some hefty effort to get my father-in-law into the seat, but once situated, Jack could remain in the chair, which then could be rolled to different rooms in the house, and Jack could be secure and kept busy for hours. Or, he would stare off to one side or doze. However, he was not always cooperative. As his dementia progressed, Jack, who formerly had been wonderfully mild-mannered, might let loose with ear-splitting invectives and uncontrolled agitation, shouting colorful and vile words that he had never spoken previously. It was embarrassing and tragic, and sadly is not uncharacteristic of more severe Alzheimer's disease patients. Most painfully troubling to me, however, at those stages of losing Jack to his disease, was that while my father-in-law would be constrained to his chair-like prison, our young toddler daughter similarly was confined to her stroller, playpen, or jumpy-chair in the very same room. And, our young daughter was exceeding my ailing father-in-law in her cognitive ability. Her soul was yearning, learning, and progressing while Jack's soul was ebbing and diminishing. It was haunting to watch their parallel abilities on opposite trajectories, at reverse junctures in their lives.

The Mishnah, also in *Pirkei Avot*, offers another compelling text that describes the periods of a lifetime, from childhood to the end of adulthood. In a text that parallels or presages a description of the flow of life by William Shakespeare in his play *As You Like It*, the Mishnah describes how a typical, paradigmatic soul progresses through the decades of life, primarily in the areas of learning and rational ability. These capacities are further reinforced by Maimonides' teaching that reason and intellect are the operations of the soul.

> He [Yehuda ben Tema] used to say, at five [one should begin the study of] Scripture; at ten, Mishnah; at thirteen [one becomes obligated in] the commandments; at fifteen [the study of] Talmud; at eighteen the wedding canopy; at twenty to pursue [a vocation]; at thirty strength; at forty understanding; at fifty counsel; at sixty old age; at seventy fullness of years; at eighty spiritual strength; at ninety bending over [beneath the weight of old age, or the grave]; at one hundred it is as if he has died and passed on and ceased from the world.
>
> —*Pirkei Avot* 5:21[2]

According to the Mishnah, one begins to learn basic material, Torah, at age five and continues to develop to more sophisticated substance and subjects at subsequent ages. Eventually, the typical person marries, pursues an occupation, and reaches maturity, at which point one is expected to teach and offer counsel. At the later stages, however, the Mishnah's text teaches that an individual commonly diminishes in ability until receding to the level and abilities roughly equivalent to childhood. Note the similarity to the closing of the famous speech by Jaques in Shakespeare's *As You Like It*:

> All the world's a stage,
> And all the men and women merely players;
> They have their exits and their entrances;
> And one man in his time plays many parts,
> His acts being seven ages. At first the infant,
> Mewling and puking in the nurse's arms;
> And then the whining school-boy. . . .
> *Last scene of all,*
> *That ends this strange eventful history,*
> *Is second childishness and mere oblivion;*
> *Sans teeth, sans eyes, sans taste, sans everything.*
>
> (Act 2, scene 7, lines 139–66, italics added)

As the Bard portrayed his seven ages of man, he also described a regression late in life. Although Jaques neglects to directly describe failing memory or cognitive impairment, he implies such losses: "mere oblivion . . . sans everything." It should not be surprising that these two powerful portraits of the human landscape, though separated by fifteen hundred years and vast cultural differences, nevertheless both describe first intellectual growth and then regression in human cognitive capacity as the normative process of living. Ultimately, although we may strongly, and rightly, fear and resist the reality of dementia in the course of life, it is all too common.

When a person regresses with Alzheimer's disease, he or she also regresses as a human soul, until the soul is gone, "sans everything." Reason and intellect, the measures of Rambam's operational soul and Shakespeare's melancholy Jaques, continue to diminish until they are gone, altogether, taking the soul with them. So it was with my grandfather and with my father-in-law. David Kohn died in 1990; Jack Bloom died in 1995, almost on his birthday. Each succumbed to the empty ending that is described in both the Mishnah and in William

Shakespeare's play. Each relinquished his soul when he could no longer strive to be human. As the Rambam taught, it would not be proper for a *nefesh* to remain without knowledge and thus not to fulfill its form.

So, what of the persons, when they and their minds are ravaged by Alzheimer's disease, and they are in a profound, severe, or late dementia stage of illness? It would be wonderful, and Pollyannaish, to maintain that they are yet and still there, stalwartly standing fast against the tide of disease. It would be Pollyannaish to claim that the outwardly familiar beings are still the lovable and approachable souls they were years earlier. And, it would be Pollyannaish to overlook the troubling symptoms—pronounced memory problems, agitation, wandering behavior, hallucinations, unsteadiness and disorientation, inability to perform basic functions, and more—and yet see the same person as before, looking out from behind the blind stare.

Ultimately, the truth is that although Alzheimer's disease may leave the body relatively intact while it takes the mind, it also takes the soul of the person. Our tradition is eminently clear: a person is far more than merely a physical, functioning creature. Rather, for a person to be a person, he or she must be ensouled—must sustain a functioning and operating inner being that bears reason and intellect. Without that, one is but a shadow; one is in a place where there is no humanity.

Sadly, such is the final result of living with, and dying from, Alzheimer's disease.

Yet, there remains the Mishnah's other verse: "strive to be a human being" (*Pirkei Avot* 2:5). Our task as caregivers, loving family members, counselors, clergy, and teachers is to follow this text of the Mishnah: *hishtadeil lih'yot ish*, "strive to be a human being." If Alzheimer's disease is that place where there is diminishing or no humanity, then the Mishnah's charge, "strive to be a human being," must fall on others who are capable of fulfilling its command.

My mother-in-law, Meye, modeled the devoted caregiver: bathing, feeding, dressing, and engaging her failing husband, Jack, and even contributing precious hours to the Alzheimer's Association, often when a respite care worker could come to spell her for a morning or an afternoon. And, she modeled the Mishnah's command. She demonstrated *striving*—not merely to *be* a human being, but on *behalf* of a human being. Such is the obligation we might derive from the Mishnah, on behalf of those with Alzheimer's disease. As the disease advances from mild to moderate to severe, the patient may be unable to strive, himself or herself, to be a human being; perhaps the patient can effectively and even unwittingly deputize those who would do so on his or her behalf.

In Hebrew, deputizing, or designating another to be your agent, is called *sh'lichut*. When you assign someone else to represent you or to be an extension of you in conducting an obligation, then upon the agent's fulfilling the deed, it is considered as if you had done so. A common example of this is when a person is about to travel to Israel, friends often give money to the traveler to take overseas to give as *tzedakah* (charitable donation) in Israel. Thus, although the traveler may directly place the money in a *tzedakah* box in Israel, Judaism accounts the credit to the original donor. This is *sh'lichut*.

As we consider the question, "What of the *person*?" with Alzheimer's disease, the concept of *sh'lichut* might be helpful. Clearly, remembering Shakespeare's description, the stages of life in the Mishnah, and the primacy of intellect and reason for an operating soul as Rambam taught, we understand that the Alzheimer's patient truly and tragically must surrender his soulful being to the sinister and capricious disease. It is a place of little or no humanity. Yet, a very real *sh'lichut* remains. Everyone who cares for and tends to the patient may be understood as striving on his or her behalf and bringing humanity to that barren, forlorn place. Each person who comforts and feeds and converses with the patient is striving on his or her behalf. And, each person who supports the tired caregiver and offers a respite and encouragement is striving to bring humanity to that place.

Yes, Alzheimer's disease may rob a person of memory, mind, ability, and even his or her soul. But, it has only a mere claim on humanity, because we learn from our text, "In a place where there is no humanity, strive to be a human being." We not only offer the surrogacy of *sh'lichut* in our caring and safeguarding family and communal memory, but we also strive to see redeeming glimpses of soul, and thus humanity, even in those whose memories Alzheimer's has robbed. Sometimes it appears on a golf course. Indeed, we rightly, and even frustratingly and sadly, may ask, "What of the person?" Again, learning from our text, I believe we ultimately find the person in our continued and enduring striving.

17

❧

Spiraling Down and Up the Staircase: The Descent of Dementia and the Ascent That Follows

ANDREW R. SKLARZ

We buried my mother just hours ago; the Jewish mourning period has barely begun. And yet, it feels as though my time as a mourner is nearing its close, not its beginning. Is the nightmare my mother and our family have been living for the last five years now over? Has redemption finally been brought to my mother's soul? Have we who loved her been liberated from the hell of her descent down the spiral staircase of dementia?

That I am writing these words in the wee hours of the night suggests that my declaration of closure might be premature. Certainly, the days, weeks, and months ahead will reveal the truth, for it is barely two days since my mother's journey on earth came to an end. Nevertheless, I feel much more at ease than I have since the onset of her illness, nearly five years ago. And though I do not feel guilty for not truly experiencing the pangs associated with mourning, I am curious as to why they are not present. Am I in denial? Have I begun the process of healing—or have I been mourning for five years already?

In the Babylonian Talmud (*Makot* 7a) we learn of the phrase *y'ridah l'tzorech aliyah*, "going way down in order to rise way up."[1] In other words, hitting rock bottom into the depths of despair may in fact catapult an individual to reach new heights.

Indeed in some instances, true growth of an individual can only occur through profound challenge and adversity. I imagine that my mother's death, a moment I dreaded, has been a moment of liberation. This final blow brought an end to the languishing sadness that I experienced throughout the duration of her illness.

I sit, musing on what has transpired since my mother's diagnosis. Previously, when I contemplated how I might feel when Mom died, my breath would stop. But surprisingly, once I bid her good-bye, I was able to breathe more freely than I had in five years. With the start of shivah, when I spoke of Mom, I could actually laugh and not cry for the first time since her diagnosis. Was this new stage in my life not quite as filled with the horror I had dreaded? Fear, sadness, and terror had gripped me from when I was first told that Mom had Alzheimer's disease, and the heartache intensified incrementally as the disease stripped my mother of nearly everything and in turn robbed us of the woman whom we loved. *Y'ridah*—it was our going down.

I will never forget the day my mother asked me my name, the name she had given me in memory of her adored grandfather. My mother, Ann, was a bright, perceptive, resourceful woman, whose life had been characterized by intellectual gifts and scholarly pursuits. As a young girl, she skipped two grades in the New York public school system, graduating at age sixteen, and subsequently graduating New York University at age nineteen. Her keen mind had defied a psychology professor's hypothesis that the human brain could memorize only a limited sequence of numbers. My mother was at first a history teacher, and her second career was as a reading and literacy specialist for underprivileged children. She was beloved by countless children who otherwise would have fallen between the cracks. Her thirst for knowledge was trumped only by her desire to instill in others a passion for learning.

* * *

A month has elapsed since that that first sleepless night, and despite a few nightmares associated with Mom's death during the week of shivah, my hunch was correct. My healing did seem to begin when I said that farewell to Mom, and I had my final cry at her grave. I believe that with my mother's death she finally achieved peace, and consequently I was able to have my own peace, too.

While this chapter will share my mother's downward spiral with dementia, her *y'ridah*, there are essentially two separate stories within it: her story and mine, and our points of intersection. As human beings, despite our relationships with other people, our journeys are nevertheless uniquely our own. This chapter, which is therapeutic for me to write as an author and hopefully therapeutic for the reader, will focus on both my mother's descent into darkness and my learning to cope with her decline and, I believe, my own spiritual rebirth, my *aliyah*, as a consequence of her demise from this dreadful illness.

As well, as I review and reflect upon both my and my mom's journeys through Alzheimer's disease, the words of the biblical Book of Jonah resonate with our experiences. Just as Jonah was cast into the turbulent sea, plummeting downwards, and then was saved and cast back upon dry land to complete his trek, so too our respective journeys have followed such a path. The biblical poet expressed the feelings that we also experienced:

> *Adonai* provided a huge fish to swallow Jonah. . . . Jonah prayed to *Adonai* . . . , saying: ". . . The waters closed in over me, the deep engulfed me, weeds twined around my head. I sank to the base of the mountains. The bars of the earth closed upon me forever. Yet, You brought me up from the pit."
> —Jonah 2:1–3, 2:6–7

Mom had always been a fiercely independent person. She kept herself in tip-top shape all her life. For years I had commented, "My mother would be dead before anyone had ever known she had been ill." Always low-key, particularly when it came to her health or personal demands from others, I was certain that one night she would go to bed, and the following morning I would receive the dreaded phone call. Well into her eighties, Mom's zest for life, her good health, and her attention to her physical appearance belied her age. On the go, traveling far, taking courses, attending study groups, and always choosing to walk, it seemed as though Mom would keep going strong indefinitely.

My parents had me later in life. My father was older than my mother and was plagued by a host of medical conditions throughout his life. He seemed to me far older than his actual years. Dad's physical decline took place over decades, and his death seemed to be a natural and expected part of his deterioration. In contrast, my mother retained her vibrancy, for the most part, until she neared her eighty-fifth birthday. Then, suddenly, old age took hold with a fury, heralded by the diagnosis of dementia. There was nothing gradual in this cruel event; one person seemed to disappear as another quickly emerged, and a dramatic physical change accompanied her mental deterioration.

After my father's death, Mom continued traveling to Florida each winter. Days before Mom's final trip, she confided to me, nonchalantly, not to be surprised if she were to die over the next months. Tears welled up in my eyes, but Mom assured me that her physician had examined her, and he felt confident about her maintaining her routine. She just felt she was slowing down. Looking back on this conversation, I realize that very compassionately, Mom wished to prepare me for something she believed would come in the near future, and she wanted the opportunity to say a loving "good-bye" to me privately. Never one for drama, bravado, attention, or sympathy, Mom merely articulated her belief that the process of aging, which seemed to have been held in abeyance, was suddenly taking its toll. She wished to soften a blow that she felt was imminent. Mom must have come to terms with the change that was occurring; she was far more on cue than the rest of us.

Yes, there had been some age-related issues I had noticed in Mom: apprehension with driving distances or driving at night, as well as comments that her bridge game wasn't up to par or that she was not as adept with the *New York Times* crossword puzzle as she had always been. In retrospect, I remember, months before her diagnosis, some increased anxiety—her frustration with a new computer and confusion with her cell phone—but I rationalized that modern technology was just posing challenges to her.

Toward her third month in Florida, Mom commented that she planned on finding a local internist, should she ever need one. There was no urgency on her part other than being prudent and practical. Weeks later, Mom had scheduled an appointment with a doctor.

> But *Adonai* cast a mighty wind upon the sea, and such a great tempest came upon the sea that the ship was in danger of breaking up.
> —Jonah 1:4

I called Mom after her appointment. With a tone of sadness that I had never heard before, Mom shared the doctor's belief that she was in the very early stages of Alzheimer's disease. My heart sank with the defeat and despair in my mother's voice—a voice that always had been positive facing any challenge. Four years earlier, when I was diagnosed with leukemia, Mom refused to accept that death would come. When I shared my diagnosis with her, Mom looked me in the eye and said, "You will not die. I won't allow it. We will find the right doctors, the right treatment, the right cure." But what could I offer my mother at the moment that she announced her diagnosis with Alzheimer's disease? While leukemia in 2006, though life-threatening, had become survivable, as of that day there was no miracle on the horizon when it came to Alzheimer's disease. The best I could offer was telling Mom that we would seek a second opinion and that Susan, the children, and I would soon come for our annual pilgrimage to Florida for her birthday. I felt a profound despair, heartbreak, and anticipation of loss.

Two days prior to her eighty-fifth birthday, we arrived in Florida, and Mom was clearly not the same woman who had left Connecticut three months earlier. Although she was still in control and capable of giving explicit and logical instructions, there was a restlessness, and a discomfort with being left alone, as well as requests for help with tasks that ordinarily she would have done herself. Independence and alone time had always been important to Mom, and she always feared having to depend on others. But that had changed. She just wasn't the quick, sharp, or composed woman I had always known. She had begun her descent.

In Florida, Mom handed over the car keys to me and said that she would not get behind the wheel again. Putting her Florida home on the market, she contacted a realtor, and we visited an independent-living facility. Mom certainly was in control, yet something was not the same.

Having made the decision to stop driving, Mom could no longer remain in her condominium in Connecticut. Thus, before her return north, my brother, Mark, found a beautiful independent-living facility for Mom. Shortly before this move, she came to spend a few days with us in Philadelphia. The physical change was dramatic. The stairs in our house became a major challenge and winded her. Walking no longer came with ease. However, the greatest shock was when suddenly she asked me my profession. Had she forgotten that I was a rabbi? Noting my astonishment, Mom lovingly commented, "Don't take it personally, dear. There is something wrong with my brain." Sadly, I needed to acknowledge that there certainly was.

A few weeks later, Mom moved into the independent-living apartment in which she would spend the final chapter of her life. It was crushing to me that my mother was now at such a stage. Most distressing was the repetition of questions regarding the move. The lengthy conversations that we had always enjoyed were no longer to be. Now, there were pregnant pauses. After seeing Mom in her new apartment, I got into my car and cried like a baby, acknowledging the beginning of the end. My period of mourning had begun. I had reached a new nadir of *y'ridah* in my journey.

> From the belly of Sheol I cried out. . . . You cast me into the depths, into the heart of the sea, the flood engulfed me; all your breakers and billows swept over me; I thought I was driven away out of your sight.
>
> —Jonah 2:3–5

When my children were born, I viewed each new development with fascination and delight, as if they were exotic flowers. Like all new parents, I reveled in their strides, the unfolding of their petals. In contrast, when one observes a dementia patient, it is as if the petals wilt each day, and one by one, shrivel up and die, then drop to the ground. Physically my mother also declined as her mind went, and the motivation to care for her body dwindled in the process. Mom, who had rapidly walked miles well into her eighties, became more and more stationary. In time, she began to depend on a walker and eventually was perfectly happy to be pushed in a wheelchair. Once when she was still walking, as we went outside for a stroll, my six-year-old son was pulling my right hand in one direction, and my mother was clinging onto my left hand for dear life. I will never forget being pulled in opposite directions by two, each so dependent upon me.

Two years after the diagnosis, our eldest child, Daniella, was to become a bat mitzvah. On the day in 1995 when Dani was born, Mom held the granddaughter for whom she had waited a lifetime and blurted out, "Oh my God, I'll be eighty-seven when Dani becomes a bat mitzvah. I might not be there!" My brother, Mark, responded, "You'll be there. We may have to wheel you in, but you'll be there." How true Mark's words came to be, but in 1995, the last thought in anyone's mind was that Mom would not be with us mentally.

I was determined that Mom would be a part of this milestone in Dani's life. Mom was our children's only surviving grandparent, and I felt it was important that she participate. For months leading up to the day, every time I spoke to Mom, I mentioned the upcoming event, hoping that details would be retained.

Nearly three hundred guests were in attendance as Dani became a bat mitzvah, including relatives, friends from my childhood and college years, and congregants who had known Mom. Would Mom recognize them, or would this be a source of frustration? Would she derive pleasure from the day, or would it be a source of embarrassment?

For sixteen years I had been a congregational rabbi, and every week, as I officiated at *b'nei mitzvah* services, I passed the Torah scroll through the generations. I wondered if my mother could participate in this ritual, or would we be deprived of this memory? When I began the service, as Dani and I stood by the pulpit, Mom gave me the same broad smile she had done for so many years. With exuberance from her front-row seat, she exclaimed to Mark, "There's Andy and there's Dani!"

Mom could not comfortably climb the steps to the bimah, hold the Torah scroll, or pass it down. Thus, I walked into the congregation and placed it into her arms for her to symbolically pass it to my daughter. Mom's smile was wide, and there was such an expression of joy on her face. I knew that I had made the right decision for Mom to participate.

While I am glad that Mom was with us for the bat mitzvah, in the pictures the look in her eyes is telling: Mom was not fully present that night. The blunt affect and sense of confusion that characterize dementia had replaced the sparkle that would have been there. In discussing his experience with cancer, Stuart Schoffman refers to S. Ansky's play, *The Dybbuk*, also known as *Between Two Worlds*, in which the phrase *y'ridah tzorech aliyah*, "going way down in order to rise way up," is spoken in the opening scene.[2] It is used as an image of being between two worlds, and indeed, my mother was in such a state. Her body was on earth, but her mind seemed to be traveling to a mysterious realm. Each day, her very essence was descending, but perhaps her soul was actually making an ascent. It was as if she was between two worlds.

Often we hear how roles are reversed for adult children with parents who are afflicted with dementia. While the dynamics of the relationship change dramatically, new dimensions, which if embraced for what they are, can bring joy for both parent and child. As my mother descended the spiral of this disease, and though painful to compare her to the woman she had been, there was a level of true peace that now was part of her new self. Much of the normal angst of living that all human beings develop as we grow was no longer part of her existence: no worries, no insecurity, no cynicism. Perhaps this is not such a terrible way to spend the last chapter of one's life. Most importantly, however, it became clear too that human beings never lose the capacity to experience love or cherish the feeling of being loved. From the moment we leave the womb until the day we die, human beings always seek love, though it may be sublimated in different forms. Along the way, our basic needs may become clouded by personal issues. There is an innocence that we find in childhood, which is later mirrored within a dementia patient, that trusts the world and is happy by the presence, attention, touch, or loving embrace of another human being.

Perhaps the sweetest dimension of my own parent-child dynamic evolved at that time, parallel perhaps to when I was a baby and Mom cared for me. The once-child was now truly becoming the self-actualized adult-child. Week after week when I would sit in Mom's room, there was such a sense of tenderness that prevailed as I sat by her, held her hand, stroked her hair, or massaged her neck, and she would respond with the word, "Delicious." Having experienced *y'ridah*, going down, I was now rebounding to *aliyah*, going up.

In her famous book *On Death and Dying*, Dr. Elisabeth Kübler-Ross outlines stages of the process of dying: denial, anger, bargaining, depression, and acceptance. Similarly, these stages also apply to one whose parent is experiencing the downward spiral of dementia. In describing her family's process with her father, Ronald Reagan, and his battle with Alzheimer's disease, Patti Davis aptly chose her mother's descriptor of the disease as the title of her book, *The Long Goodbye*, addressing "the way in which Alzheimer's steals away a person."[3] While I concur, I also celebrate that within this process I gained new insights into myself, discovering ultimately how I have grown through partnering with my mother as she traveled this road. While some might call her illness a tragic end to a vital life, Mom's epilogue was peaceful and, as I reflect upon it, perhaps was a perfect way to move on to God.

From the time of Mom's diagnosis, I had been awaiting the call that Mom had died or was on the brink of death. Yet, on another level, my fear was that the call might not be soon enough—not because I wished for Mom to die, but because I feared her coming to the point in which she would be robbed of everything. Fortunately, that never happened. When I spoke to her the day before her death, though she needed to be told, "It's Andy, your son," Mom was bright, cheerful, and thankful for my call. I ended every conversation during her illness with the words, "I love you, Mom," and she responded in kind.

Then, one night, Mom suffered a massive stroke, and there was no brain activity. It was time for her to go.

When Mark reached me that night from the emergency room, he put the phone to Mom's ear so I could say "good-bye," tell her I loved her one last time, and encourage her to move on to God. The next morning, minutes before I arrived at her hospital room, Mom passed. Perhaps her spirit knew it was time to move forward.

That afternoon, I went to Mom's apartment for the last time. The walls were filled with photos from the nearly ten decades of her life. I remembered Mom speaking about the joys and challenges in her life. She had commented, "The pluses outweigh the minuses, and I've had a lot of fun."

The sad pictures in my mind of the last five years have given way to the many happy pictures, both actual and those in memory, of the mother I had known for forty-six years. Mom's epilogue, with the exception of the joy I believe we experienced during my visits, has faded in my mind. I no longer think of the experience as a "nightmare." I no longer ask, "What happened to my mother—that smart and savvy woman?" The wonderful pictures have entered the forefront of my mind when I think of Mom.

> You brought me my life from the pit, O *Adonai* my God!
> When my life was ebbing away, I called *Adonai* to mind;
> And my prayer came before You, into Your holy temple. . . .
> Deliverance is *Adonai*'s.
>
> —Jonah 2:7–8, 2:10

After writing the first paragraphs of this chapter in the wee hours of the morning following the first night of shivah, I waited until after the period of *sh'loshim* (thirty days) had concluded before I continued my writing. My hunch was correct. While there has not been a day that I haven't thought of Mom, there is no sense of acute sadness. Do I miss the woman who had been my mother prior to the illness? Would I like to give a hug and receive a loving smile from that kind lady who could not quite remember the name she had given me but nevertheless was happy to see me? Yes; however, I am at peace, and I believe that Mom is now truly at peace. From a *y'ridah* came an *aliyah*.

> Bestow Your favor on us, O *Adonai*. . . .
> Safe and sound—*in peace*, I lie down and sleep.
>
> —Psalm 4:7, 4:9[4]

18

The Whole World Is Full of God's Glory

CARY KOZBERG

I

Do not cast me off in the time of old age; forsake me not when my strength fails me.

(Psalm 71:9)

I often think of this verse when I see visitors come into our nursing home. If they are "first-timers"—if their loved one has not resided here for a long time, or if they are relatively uninformed about what we do and how and why we do it—their facial expressions often echo the fear of growing old and becoming frail expressed by the Psalmist's words. Sometimes, if they are self-aware and honest, they may even articulate their fear and the profound sense of helplessness that creeps up on them when they come through our doors.

But even when their feelings remain unexpressed, one only has to look into their eyes in order to know that they believe they are in the "valley of the shadow of death" (Psalm 23:4). So stark is the "otherness" of this place that the proverbial comfort of "Your rod and Your staff" (ibid.) may well elude them. They have come into a place where failed strength and damaged faculties are acknowledged realities for residents and frightening possibilities for visitors. Viewed as "holding areas" for the Angel of Death, nursing homes are places that most people instinctively avoid.

And no other places in a nursing home seem to broadcast this message more clearly than where people with advanced dementia reside. A visit to a dementia-designated floor (or "neighborhood") on any given day, at any given hour, is a visit to a foreign land—another world where language, the rules for communication and socialization, and the reference points of "reality" are completely different.

Not only are the inhabitants of this land pitied, they often are viewed as less than human. Living in a "hypercognitive" culture (to use Stephen Post's felicitous adjective),[1] a culture that values a person's worth based on his or her mental acuity, we often assume that when a person's cognitive functioning decreases, so does his or her worth as a human being. It is as if the Cartesian declaration, "I think, therefore I am," had an axiomatic obverse: "If I no longer think, I no longer am." Unfortunately, such a conclusion all too commonly leads to an assumption that individuals with advanced dementia are less than human. Moreover, it also has led to advocacy by some philosophers and ethicists for an ethical model that *narrows* the definition of "personhood" to exclude those with advanced dementia.

In this exclusionary model, those without certain "operative capacities"—self-awareness, self-control, a sense of the future and the past, as well as other capacities that persons with dementia eventually lose—would fall outside the definition of "personhood." Without these capacities, they no longer would be entitled to the full moral and legal protection that accompanies being a full "person," not to mention the resources now expended to care for them.[2]

Moreover, as their capacities diminish and they face becoming virtually inanimate, unable to do anything on their own, they are often described and defined by another word, one that takes away any remaining vestige of their humanity: "vegetable."

Of course, Judaism (as well as Christianity and Islam) affirms that every human being, no matter how capable or compromised, is created in the divine image and therefore is sacred and has infinite, unconditional worth. Thus, the belief that a human being could ever *not* be "fully human," much less a "vegetable," is not a Jewish point of view. Indeed, Jewish tradition teaches that even a *goseis*—a person who is actively dying—is still fully human and may not even be touched, lest death be hastened. For those of us who are concerned not only with "quality of life" but also with its *sanctity*, we associate using the "V" word with using the "N" word when referring to African Americans: it is not just politically incorrect, it is a sacrilege.

In my role as rabbi and chaplain of a Jewish senior residential care facility, I bear witness to Judaism's affirmation of the sanctity of life, to the truth that frail and compromised people are still human, and to its corollary that despite their compromises, they too have spiritual needs. Over the years, I have spent countless hours in the land of advanced dementia, helping residents to stay spiritually and culturally connected to God, Torah, and the Jewish people through whatever capacities they still may retain. In playing to their strengths, I've come to learn that *cognitive* impairment is not the same as, nor does it necessarily imply, *spiritual* impairment. Indeed, I've had the privilege of meeting many cognitively impaired individuals who appear to be much more spiritually attuned than many who are more cognitively intact. Serving residents with dementia, who often receive only our pity, I am always inspired by the midrash that teaches how every person present at Sinai heard God's Voice, according to his or her own abilities. Everyone heard it uniquely, because the Voice was heard not only by the mind, but also by the soul.

One individual who continued to hear the Voice until his dying day was a gentleman whom I will call Joe.

Joe was a resident on our dementia neighborhood[3] coping with advanced Alzheimer's disease. As his cognitive abilities waned, he forgot the words to the blessing over the wine, and his responses didn't always fit the question he was asked. But for all of his limitations, I could always count on him to help set the right atmosphere for our weekly *Kabbalat Shabbat* (welcoming the Sabbath) program in the neighborhood. He would always greet me with a warm handshake, a smile, and a reminder: "Rabbi, it's time to talk to the Boss!" In his inimitable way, Joe helped create a *Shabbesdik* (Sabbath-filled) atmosphere for everyone present. Even with all of the losses he had sustained—loss of memory, loss of executive function, loss of bowel and bladder control—he was one of the most spiritually attuned people I've ever met, continuing to pray and sing with joyful enthusiasm and heartfelt spontaneity at every opportunity.

To be sure, most of us hope we will never be in Joe's place. Indeed, as products of a hypercognitive culture, many of us believe that dementia not only would rob us of our ability to remember and think and independently engage in the normal activities of daily living, it also would rob us of our personhood, and therefore of any reason to go on living. Such is the fear behind the directive I've heard so often: "If I ever get to be that way, just take me out and shoot me!"

And yet, having worked with people like Joe, I have seen how Alzheimer's disease actually can be a boon to their "personhood," precisely, and ironically, because it is a boon to their spirituality. I have seen how feelings of joy, spontaneity, enthusiasm, and gratitude are actually heightened in a person with dementia, because those feelings no longer pass through the cognitive filter of the rational mind. I continue to marvel at how folks like Joe actually seem more fortunate than those of us who still have that filter. With the loss of cognition and memory, they no longer worry about the past or the future. Living only in the present, they usually are more at ease and will respond to those who show them affection and a caring attitude. One might say that because of their loss of the filter of reason and self-consciousness, they are able to trust more readily.

To be sure, "trust" may not be the most appropriate word here. Certainly theirs is not a trust that emerges from conscientious or cognitive choice, for the disease process itself has forced a surrender of their ability to conscientiously choose anything. But when offered love, compassion, and physical contact, they respond with feelings of assurance and affection that are more intuitive, more primal . . . and more pure. Indeed, when they are no longer aware that they are no longer aware, they give themselves over—sometimes all too enthusiastically—to the faithful care of others, whether human or divine.

Eventually (and sadly), folks like Joe usually lose their ability to speak and communicate cogently, and this "operative capacity" often is replaced with repetitive questioning and/or words that make little or no sense. For many with advanced dementia, the common *lingua franca* will be grunting, bleating, yelling, or sometimes just remaining in a mute stupor. But to my mind, what is even sadder is that, feeling helpless as we look upon their frailties and listen to their pathetic sounds, we usually dismiss them as lost, useless, and less than human. With pity, but without shame, we often so wrongly label them with the "V" word, "vegetables."

II

Personally, I prefer to believe that such persons are more like *angels*, and I have had this belief for twenty-two years—ever since my first day on the job, when I moved into my office that was adjacent to our dementia neighborhood. I remember telling myself at the time that the sounds emanating from "this other world" would have little effect on me.

I was so wrong.

Having left my door open on that first day, I soon discovered that the grunting and the gibberish that came out of that area were sounds like the odor of incontinence—an expected but unavoidable part of the environment to which one—I—must become accustomed. Yet, the more I became accustomed, the more I understood that in this part of the world these sounds are not just to be expected, but in a curious but significant way they are actually needed. My mind went to the words that are recited daily in the traditional *Shacharit* (morning) service:

> They [the Heavenly Beings] all perform with awe and reverence the will of their Creator; they all open their mouths with holiness and purity . . . with pure speech and sacred melody, they all exclaim in unison and with reverence:

> Holy, holy, holy is *Adonai Tseva'ot*; the whole world is full of His glory.[4]

Our Sages teach that when we recite the *K'dushah* prayer and proclaim God's sanctity in the world, just as the angels did in Isaiah's vision (Isaiah 6:2–3), we create a "symmetry of sanctity" with these heavenly beings. Just as angels were created to continually praise God, human beings were created for the same reason. Though no longer vibrant, active individuals with intact "operative capacities," individuals with dementia are like angels; like angels, they do not consciously choose to praise God as the rest of us do, they do it automatically, as we declare every Shabbat morning, "The breath of *every* living thing will bless Your name" (italics mine).[5]

People with dementia are like angels in another important way: they too are perhaps unwitting "messengers from God." The message they deliver is a standing invitation from the Creator beckoning us to reflect upon what it means to be human. They charge us to be grateful for our God-given gifts and abilities, but also to know what their limitations are; to discern when we must take responsibility for our lives, and when to realize when we must "let go" and put our trust in others—again, whether human or divine.

One of the reasons it is hard to be in the presence of these individuals is because the message they bring is difficult or painful for us to hear. We live in a culture that promotes independence and self-reliance, and to avoid being dependent and relying on others. We hope (more accurately: expect) to be in control of our life circumstances until the moment we die. For some people, the very notion of "trust" itself presents challenges, and thus they endeavor to remain self-reliant at all costs. Perhaps they have been betrayed too many times, and cynicism has taken root in their souls. Even when we affirm the importance of trusting others, we may still shy away from the risk of "letting go" and surrendering our "selves" to others. Such a deep skepticism is not new to Jews, nor is it just a result of secularism and the challenges of modernity. On the contrary, this widespread skepticism is part of our collective Jewish psyche, dating to a distrust of God repeatedly shown by our ancestors who left Egypt. As Torah narratives repeatedly recount, although witnessing firsthand a miraculous redemption that affirmed God's covenantal commitment, our ancestors never abandoned their doubts of God's love for them. Despite everything they saw, they still could not "let go" and surrender their future to their Divine Benefactor. For this reason, they earned for themselves the epithet "stiff-necked people" (Exodus 32:9).

We, their descendants, are no less "stiff-necked." In such a culture, we Jews will continue to pity folks like Joe and even consider them less than full "persons." We may even dispassionately and without shame refer to them with the "V" word. But we who work with the Joes of this world see them less as victims to be pitied and more as teachers, albeit unwitting, offering critical and substantive lessons to be heeded.

Daily, they teach us that life can still be edifying and even purposeful, even in the face of losses and limitations caused by dementia. Daily, they remind us that these losses and limitations are themselves limited: they are powerless to diminish the spontaneous and genuine love and joy that people with dementia can still experience, which also may testify to an abiding godliness in their lives. Daily, they teach us that in the midst of coping with what many view as a curse, they not only receive but in turn give back blessings that have nothing to do with "operative capacities." Daily, they remain angelic.

III

I am aware that despite my having described persons with dementia as angelic, many will remain unconvinced. While they may concede that persons with dementia are not dead nor are they "vegetables," neither are they prepared to see them as fully alive; they are more "in between." But even if this is so, we would do well to remember the observation of Martin Buber: it is the spaces "in between" where reality resides and thus where one encounters holiness.[6]

Ultimately, our perspective on persons with dementia depends on how we choose to see and interpret. We can choose to hear the grunts, shrieks, and bleating as cacophonies of suffering and of abandonment in seemingly "God-forsaken" places. Or we can choose to understand them as sacred and "God-filled," in and of themselves. If the whole world truly *is* full of God's glory, then even these places, seemingly filled with helplessness and death, cannot truly be "God-forsaken." The sounds that are emitted from such persons in such places are the very lyrics of this testimony.

Curiously, we humans not only revere "the holy," but also avoid it. We experience the sacred not only with awe and reverence, but also with fear (significantly, the Hebrew word *yirah* denotes both meanings, "fear" and "reverence," simultaneously). This is the nature of the "numinous." Mysteriously filled with divinity, it is also somehow taboo: it is sacrosanct and too risky to encounter. As Sam Keen has observed:

> In the life of the spirit, paradox is the rule . . . the opposites coincide, the diseased parts form a graceful whole. . . . In considering the whole and holiness of life, we must at once hold before our eyes visions of horror and wonder, cruelty and kindness. . . . Both/ and, not either/or.[7]

My continuing prayer is that when we are in the presence of people with advanced dementia, we will come to know on a deeper level that, even in the "valley of the shadow," the comfort of God's "rod and staff" abides and is ever present and that we may actually have angels in our midst. With this in mind, may we understand that our fear and avoidance with such people may be as much due to an abiding tension with sanctity that is both present and taboo as they are due to the painful deterioration and debilitation that seem so tangibly evident.

Discerning this, may we know why human beings—especially those with advanced dementia—will always *be* human. Discerning this, may we affirm anew that "the whole world *is* full of God's glory," even when the world is broken. And may we merit the ability to glue the broken fragments back together and ultimately, redeem them.

Biographies

RABBI RICHARD F. ADDRESS, DMin, serves as senior rabbi of Congregation M'kor Shalom in Cherry Hill, New Jersey. Previously, he served the Union for Reform Judaism and was the founding director of the Department of Jewish Family Concerns. In that capacity he helped develop the award-winning program on Sacred Aging, which stressed the spiritual development of baby boomers. He received his DMin in 1999 from Hebrew Union College–Jewish Institute of Religion and continues to teach in that program. Rabbi Address is also the editor of Jewish Sacred Aging (jewishsacredaging.com), has edited several books dealing with Judaism and aging, and writes for websites on the subject. He is the author of *Seekers of Meaning: Baby Boomers, Judaism, and the Pursuit of Healthy Aging* (URJ Press).

RONALD M. ANDIMAN, MD, is clinical chief of neurology at Cedars-Sinai Medical Center, Los Angeles, and director of its inpatient management program. He is clinical professor of neurology at the Keck

School of Medicine, University of Southern California. He has been in the private practice of neurology for thirty-one years and sees a broad spectrum of neurological problems. After graduating from the Albert Einstein College of Medicine, he did his internship at Boston City Hospital, residency at the Mount Sinai Hospital, New York City, and a fellowship in neuromuscular disease at UCLA. After serving on the full-time faculty at USC for five years, he went into private practice and during that period, for over twenty years, spent part of his time as the rehabilitation director of a local community hospital. Dr. Andiman has read a poem with his rehabilitation staff at each of the weekly patient management conferences for a number of years. He is married and has three daughters and three grandchildren.

RABBI MIKE COMINS is the founder of the TorahTrek Center for Jewish Wilderness Spirituality and the author of *A Wild Faith: Jewish Ways into Wilderness, Wilderness Ways into Judaism* and *Making Prayer Real: Leading Jewish Spiritual Voices on Why Prayer Is Difficult and What to Do about It*. He studied classical Jewish texts for four years at the Pardes Institute, earned his MA in Jewish education from Hebrew University, and was ordained in the Israeli rabbinical program of Hebrew Union College–Jewish Institute of Religion. Finding his calling in life, Rabbi Comins became a licensed desert guide and led wilderness retreats in Israel and the Sinai. He founded TorahTrek while serving the Jewish Community of Jackson Hole, Wyoming. Living in Los Angeles with his wife, Jody, he writes, teaches, and leads wilderness programs throughout North America.

RABBI ELLIOT N. DORFF, PhD, is rector and distinguished professor of philosophy at the American Jewish University in Los Angeles and visiting professor at UCLA School of Law. He is chair of the Conservative Movement's Committee on Jewish Law and Standards and a past president of Jewish Family Service of Los Angeles. Rabbi Dorff is the author of over two hundred articles on Jewish thought, law, and ethics, editor or coeditor of fourteen books on those topics, and author of twelve more. His book *Matters of Life and Death: A Jewish Approach to Modern Medical Ethics* discusses some issues related to the topic of his essay in this book.

CANTOR ELLEN DRESKIN is an innovative leader in today's Reform Movement. Her expertise extends from contemporary Jewish music to synagogue transformation, from experiential education to enlivened liturgy and Jewish mysticism. She currently serves as coordinator of the Cantorial Certification Program at the Debbie Friedman School of Sacred Music at Hebrew Union College–Jewish Institute of Religion in New York. Cantor Dreskin has served as cantor and educator for congregations in Cleveland and New York, travels extensively to congregations around the country as a scholar-in-residence, and has taught for many years on the faculty of URJ Summer Kallot, Hava Nashira, and the URJ Kutz Camp Leadership Academy. She is married to Rabbi Billy Dreskin and is the proud mother of Katherine Elizabeth, Jonah Maccabee (*z''l*), and Aiden Madison.

BEVERLY L. ENGEL has nearly thirty years' experience in the field of aging, guiding organizations through the visualization, creation, and implementation of programs that promote health and well-being for elders and caregivers. With an MS in gerontology from the Leonard Davis School of Gerontology at the University of Southern California, an MA in Jewish communal service from Hebrew Union College–Jewish Institute of Religion, and a BA from Douglass College, Rutgers University, Engel has worked in academic, hospital, and community-based arenas and with a private foundation. She has designed and implemented innovative training and educational programs in geriatrics, conceived of and managed an adult day health center, and now serves the Alzheimer's Association, Central and North Florida Chapter, as program coordinator, where she is also responsible for community education efforts. Her newest initiative involves the promotion of brain-healthy lifestyles in Central Florida. Considering herself fortunate to be married to Rabbi Steven Engel and the mother of three adult children, Engel also wholeheartedly embraces her role as daughter to her parents and in-laws.

MINA FRIEDLER has been using poetry, art, and music to construct creative programs that stimulate memory for seniors and seniors with dementias for more than twenty years throughout the Los Angeles area. She received a BA in political science from University of California, Berkeley in 1982 and a JD from Southwestern University in 1986. However, she discovered her true calling, working with seniors, in 1989, shortly after her marriage to Dr. Eli Friedler, a geriatric psychiatrist, when they spent an amazing Rosh HaShanah blowing the shofar and visiting elderly, sick patients near Chabad of Santa Monica. When Friedler touched the hands of the needy, she felt so much love and connectedness that she knew she wanted to serve them for the rest of her life. She recently became director of the Jewish Family Service Israel Levin Center, a senior community center in Venice, California. She lives in Venice with her husband, and she eats lunch on the sands next to the waves of the Pacific Ocean, gazing at the horizon and up at the blue skies.

RABBI ELYSE GOLDSTEIN served for twenty years as the director of Kolel in Toronto. She is currently creating a new Reform congregation in downtown Toronto. She graduated summa cum laude and Phi Beta Kappa from Brandeis University in 1978 and received her doctor of divinity, honoris causis, from Brandeis in 2008. She writes a monthly column for the *Canadian Jewish News* and is one of seven women featured in the Canadian National Film Board documentary *Half the Kingdom*. Rabbi Goldstein is the author of *ReVisions: Seeing Torah through a Feminist Lens* and *Seek Her Out: A Textual Approach to the Study of Women and Judaism* (URJ Press) and editor of *The Women's Torah Commentary*, *The Women's Haftarah Commentary*, and *New Jewish Feminism: Probing the Past, Forging the Future*.

RABBI PAUL J. KIPNES leads Congregation Or Ami in Calabasas, California. Under his leadership, Or Ami has won national awards for social justice programming, innovative worship, outreach to interfaith families, engaging family education, and use of technology in a synagogue. He also creates community-wide programs for Jews recovering from addictions. He is coediting a national *CCAR Journal* issue on "New Visions for Jewish Community." Rabbi Kipnes teaches pastoral counseling in the Rabbinical School at Hebrew Union College–Jewish Institute of Religion, serves on the clinical faculty of the Rhea Hirsch School of Jewish Education, and is rabbinic dean at Camp Newman in Santa Rosa, California, and chair of the Revenue Enhancement Committee of the Central Conference of American Rabbis. He blogs at http://rabbipaul.blogspot.com and tweets @RabbiKip. A fan of meditation, *Star Trek*, and yoga, Rabbi Kipnes and his wife, Michelle November, have three children.

RABBI DOUGLAS J. KOHN became rabbi of Southern California's oldest synagogue, Redland's historic Congregation Emanu El, in 2001, after serving synagogues in Buffalo, Baltimore, and Chicago. An Antioch College and Hebrew Union College–Jewish Institute of Religion graduate, he is concerned about social justice and Israel and has served on the Commission on Social Action of Reform Judaism and the national board of the Association of Reform Zionists of America (ARZA). He was a delegate to the opening of the Mychoels Jewish Center in Moscow in 1989 and to the World Zionist Congress in 2006. Rabbi Kohn is the editor of *Life, Faith, and Cancer: Jewish Journeys through Diagnosis, Treatment and Recovery* (URJ Press) and a contributor to *World Religions for Healthcare Professionals*. An avid runner until his cancer diagnosis in 2004, now he just jogs with his two dogs. He is married to Reva Bloom and is the father of Benjamin and Elena.

RABBI CARY KOZBERG has served as director of religious life at Wexner Heritage Village in Columbus, Ohio, since 1989, developing religious and spiritual programs for Jewish and non-Jewish residents, their families, and WHV staff. He is past chair of the Forum on Religion, Spirituality, and Aging and has written and lectured extensively on the spiritual challenges facing older adults and their families. He is the author of *Honoring Broken Tablets: A Jewish Approach to Dementia* and coeditor (with Rabbi James Michaels) of *Flourishing in The Later Years: Jewish Pastoral Insights on Senior Residential Care*. Rabbi Kozberg is the recipient of the National Association of Jewish Chaplains 2012 "Chaplain of the Year" award. In his spare time, he enjoys his family, his dogs, and playing drums in a rock band.

TOBY F. LAPING, PhD, LMSW, opened her geriatric care management firm in Buffalo, New York, over thirty years ago. In addition, she has held appointments on the faculties of the Social Work School and Medical School Division of Geriatrics at State University of New York at Buffalo, as well as numerous consultative positions. For the past six years, she has written a monthly column in a regional newspaper focused on the senior market, and she has lectured and been published on issues related to guardianships in New York State. She recently became an incorporator of a nonprofit, aging-in-place organization called Canopy of Neighbors, designed to make it easier for seniors in her community to remain in their homes as they age. Dr. Laping is married to John, her college sweetheart, and is the mother of two children and grandmother of six.

CATHY M. LIEBLICH, MA, is special projects and coalitions coordinator for Pioneer Network. She is liaison between Pioneer Network and the thirty-eight state culture change coalitions and coordinates some grant-funded projects. She has over thirty years of experience in aging and long-term care with the National Council on the Aging, a long-term care provider association, an area agency on aging, a university center on aging, and a private foundation. Lieblich was the founding director of the Florida Pioneer Network and currently serves on the coalition's steering committee. She also serves as secretary of the board of directors of the Centers for Excellence in Assisted Living (CEAL) and on the board of the Advancing Excellence LTC Collaborative. She earned an MS in social service administration from the University of Chicago in 1980 and a BA in anthropology from the Johns Hopkins University in 1978.

RABBI SHELDON MARDER serves the Jewish Home of San Francisco, where he provides spiritual care for older adults with serious illness, end-of-life care, and Jewish pastoral care for people with dementia. His most recent articles are "God Is in the Text: Using Sacred Text and Teaching in Jewish Pastoral Care" and "Psalms, Songs & Stories: Music and Midrash at the Jewish Home of San Francisco"; his Torah teachings appear in *Voices of Torah: A Treasury of Rabbinic Gleanings on the Weekly Portions* (CCAR Press). Rabbi Marder is a coeditor and translator of the upcoming new Reform High Holy Day *machzor* (CCAR Press). He was ordained by Hebrew Union College–Jewish Institute of Religion in 1978.

RABBI MICHELE BRAND MEDWIN received a BS with honors from Cornell University in 1976 and a doctor of optometry degree from the Pennsylvania College of Optometry in 1980. After thirteen years in private practice, she was inspired to become a rabbi. She was ordained by Hebrew Union College–Jewish Institute of Religion, New York, in 1997 and has served synagogues in Broomall, Pennsylvania, and Binghamton, New York. She is currently the rabbi of Temple Sholom in Monticello, New York. She also works as a spiritual advisor for Jewish troubled teens at the Family Foundation School in Hancock, New York. Rabbi Medwin is the author of *A Spiritual Travel Guide to the World of God*. She is married to Steven Medwin and is the mother of Rabbi Dan Medwin and Rachel Witriol, Esq., mother-in-law of Rabbi Lydia Medwin and Michael Witriol, and the grandmother of Zimra.

RABBI JONATHAN V. PLAUT, DHL, DD, LLD, received his ordination in 1970 from Hebrew Union College–Jewish Institute of Religion, Cincinnati, where he earned a doctor of Hebrew letters in 1977. He served Congregation Beth El in Windsor, Ontario, from 1970 to 1984, and was the senior rabbi at Temple Emanu-El in San Jose, California, from 1985 to 1993. Returning to the Detroit area in 1993 to be closer to his children and ailing parents, Rabbi Plaut became engaged in many nonprofit fund-raising projects as well as serving congregations needing part-time rabbinic services. He led Congregation Beth El in Traverse City, Michigan, from 1999 to 2004, where he was rabbi emeritus, and since 2000 was rabbi of Temple Beth Israel in Jackson, Michigan. He authored *The Jews of Windsor 1790–1990: A Historical Chronicle*. A driving force in many civic and religious organizations during his career, Rabbi Plaut and his wife, Carol, have two married children and two grandsons.

RHONNA SHATZ, DO, joined the staff of Henry Ford Hospital in Detroit, Michigan, in 1990 as director of behavioral neurology and in 2011 was appointed as the Clayton Alandt Endowed Chair of Behavioral Neurology. She combines a passion for language and neuroscience into a vehicle for recasting the myths of dementia into advocacy for brain health. She served as cochair of Health Services Subcommittee Michigan Dementia Plan; chaired the board of directors of the Alzheimer's Association, Greater Michigan Chapter, and Medical and Scientific Advisory Council; and nurtures the spiritual aspects of medicine through Project Chesed, the Kalsman Institute, and the Adat Shalom Physician Journey group. In addition to National Institutes of Health (NIH)–funded research on Alzheimer's genetics, Dr. Shatz received a Picker Foundation grant to pilot partnerships between Alzheimer's Association, NIH cognitive Toolbox, and primary care physicians to empower their ability to diagnose and treat dementia. Every morning she runs, trying to keep up with her husband and their dogs, a Great Dane, and an Irish wolfhound.

RABBI ANDREW R. SKLARZ, MSW, became rabbi of Greenwich Reform Synagogue in 2008 after serving congregations in suburban New York and Philadelphia. He received a BA from Clark University, rabbinic ordination from Hebrew Union College–Jewish Institute of Religion, and an MSW from Fordham University. A rabbi, social worker, and psychotherapist, he is devoted to spiritual counseling, social action, and interfaith work. Years before his diagnosis of leukemia in 2001, Rabbi Sklarz served as a pastoral counselor at Memorial Sloan-Kettering Cancer Center in New York and has volunteered in hospital settings throughout his rabbinate. He was featured in the video documentary *The Journey: A Survivor's Story* and has authored chapters in volumes including *Jewish Relational Care A–Z: We Are Our Other's*

Keepers and *Life, Faith, and Cancer: Jewish Journeys through Diagnosis, Treatment, and Recovery* (URJ Press). A lover of theater, music, the arts, yoga, and cycling, he resides in Greenwich, Connecticut, with his wife, Susan, and their children, Daniella and Alexander.

RABBI BONNIE ANN STEINBERG was ordained by Hebrew Union College–Jewish Institute of Religion, New York, in 1979. A graduate of Brandeis University, she has worked at Hofstra University in Hillel, at Temple Isaiah of Great Neck, and at Temple Beth El of Huntington, New York. Since 2000, she has been the director of religious life at the Jewish Home Lifecare in the Bronx, New York. She has a certificate in bioethics and is a master's degree student in the bioethics program of Montefiore/Einstein. After growing up in Boston, Massachusetts, Rabbi Steinberg now lives in New Hyde Park on Long Island, New York, with her husband, psychologist Daniel Gensler, and their two sons, Joshua and Micah.

RABBI SIMKHA Y. WEINTRAUB, LCSW, a rabbi and social worker, serves as rabbinic director of the Jewish Board of Family and Children's Services in New York City and is centrally involved in the agency's New York Jewish Healing Center and National Center for Jewish Healing programs. He teaches pastoral skills at the Jewish Theological Seminary, is a founding board member of Rabbis for Human Rights–North America, and maintains a private practice in couples/family therapy in New York. His books include *Healing of Soul, Healing of Body* and *Guide Me Along the Way: A Jewish Spiritual Companion for Surgery*, in addition to many articles and chapters related to Jewish spiritual care and mental health. Married to Simha Rosenberg, Rabbi Weintraub is the father of Adin and Meirav.

Notes

꙳꙳

All quotes from the Torah come from *The Torah: A Modern Commentary*, revised edition, edited by W. Gunther Plaut (New York: URJ Press, 2005). Except as noted, quotes from other books of the Bible come from *The Tanakh: A New Translation of the Holy Scriptures* (Philadelphia: Jewish Publication Society, 1985).

Foreword

1. Meyer Waxman, *History of Jewish Literature* (New York: Bloch Publishing Co., 1930–1941), vol. 4, p. 612.
2. "Violin Concerto," *New York Times*, October 4, 1953.

Preface

1. Alzheimer's Association, *2011 Alzheimer's Disease Facts and Figures* (Chicago: Alzheimer's Association, 2011), p. 12.; Patricia B. Smith, Mary Mitchell Kenan, and Mark Edwin Kunik, *Alzheimer's for Dummies* (Hoboken, NJ: Wiley Publishing, Inc., 2004), p. 9.
2. *2011 Alzheimer's Disease Facts and Figures*, pp. 14, 17, 29.; Smith, Kenan, Kunik, p. 29.

Chapter 1: Normal Forgetfulness, or . . .

1. Michael S. Sweeney, *Brain: The Complete Mind* (Washington, DC: National Geographic Society, 2009), p. 95.
2. See Alzheimer's Association, www.alz.org.
3. See article by Malcolm Goldsmith, Rector of St. Cuthbert's Episcopal Church in Edinburgh, addressing the challenge dementia poses to theology, at http://www.guildofstraphael.org.uk/topics-dementia.htm.
4. Tom Kitwood, *Dementia Reconsidered: The Person Comes First* (Philadelphia: Open University Press, 1977).

Chapter 2: Recognizing Changes

1. "Chazak v'Ematz." W. Gunther Plaut, Canadian. Published in the *Canadian Jewish News*, December 11, 2003.

Chapter 3: Remember Grandma Esther

1. http://www.reocities.com/HotSprings/3004/thewatcher.html
2. http://www.werner-saumweber.de/alzheimer/poems/wanam.htm
3. Babylonian Talmud (*Menahot* 99a)
4. http://werner-saumweber.de/alzheimer/poems/forlove.htm

Chapter 4: Early Responses: Talking to Dementia with Its Own, New Language

1. Maimonides, *Sefer HaMada* 5:7.
2. I appreciate the assistance of Rabbi Douglas Kohn, who contributed this and subsequent sections incorporating the texts of Moses Maimonides.
3. Maimonides, *Shemonah Perakim: A Treatise on the Soul*, trans. Leonard S. Kravitz and Kerry M. Olitzky (New York: URJ Press, 1999), pp. 49–50.
4. Maimonides, *Sefer HaMada* 6:3.

Chapter 5: Questions of Legal Competency

1. Julius Preuss, *Biblical and Talmudic Medicine*, trans. Fred Rosner (New York: Sanhedrin Press, 1978), chap. 11. Fred Rosner, *Medicine in the Bible and the Talmud* (New York: Ktav, 1977), p. 32, classifies Saul as suffering from "paranoid psychopathia." See M. Gorlin, "Mental Illness in Biblical Literature," *Proceedings of the Association of Orthodox Jewish Scientists* 1 (1970): 43–62.
2. Babylonian Talmud, *Chagigah* 3b–4a; see also *Tosefta, T'rumot* 1:3; Babylonian Talmud, *Shabbat* 105b; *Sanhedrin* 65b; *Niddah* 17a.
3. Maimonides, *Mishneh Torah*, Laws of Testimony 9:9–11, and see the commentary of the *Kesef Mishneh* there.
4. Moshe Halevi Spero, *Judaism and Psychology: Halakhic Perspectives* (New York: Ktav, 1980), p. 175.
5. *Mishnah Chagigah* 1:1; *Mishnah Bava Kama* 8:4; Babylonian Talmud, *Gittin* 23a; *Shulchan Aruch, Choshen Mishpat* 188:2.
6. See Spero, *Judaism and Psychology*, chap. 9, pp. 120–41.
7. See I Samuel 10:5–12, 19:8–24.
8. *Tosefta, T'rumot* 1:3; see also Babylonian Talmud, *Rosh HaShanah* 28a; *Y'vamot* 31a, 113b; *K'tubot* 20a. On all of these legal ramifications, cf. Spero, *Judaism and Psychology*, chaps. 3, 9, 11, and 12.
9. Babylonian Talmud, *Rosh HaShanah* 28a; Babylonian Talmud, *Y'vamot* 113b.
10. Maimonides, *Mishneh Torah*, Laws of Testimony 9:9.
11. Babylonian Talmud, *Y'vamot* 31a–31b, 113b.
12. Ibid.

13. Babylonian Talmud, *K'tubot* 20a.

14. Babylonian Talmud, *Y'vamot* 31a. In the Rabbinic mind, the acts of be-trothal and buying were similar, for a man actually acquires a wife from her father when the groom betroths her, and the groom therefore engages in a symbolic act of *kinyan*, "acquisition," just as he would if he were acquiring real estate. This, of course, is objectionable to many moderns, and various people in the Conservative, Reconstructionist, and Reform Movements have sought to change Jewish marriage rites so that they no longer embody this parallelism to acquiring property—or at least to make the acquisition mutual.

15. Babylonian Talmud, *P'sachim* 78b.

16. Babylonian Talmud, *Bava Kama* 87a; cf. Babylonian Talmud, *Gittin* 22b.

17. *Mishnah Bava Kama* 8:4.

18. The phrase "the duress [*ones*] of sleep" is used in Babylonian Talmud, *B'rachot* 4b and is applied to criminal acts. Sleeping people are nevertheless re-sponsible for civil damages they cause (*Mishnah Bava Kama* 2:6).

19. Maimonides, *Mishneh Torah*, Laws of Evidence 9:9; *Shulchan Aruch, Choshen Mishpat* 35:9.

20. *Mishneh LaMelech* to *Mishneh Torah*, Laws of Evidence 11:8. The subject there is a woman, but the same reasoning would apply to insane men.

21. Babylonian Talmud, *Sanhedrin* 74a–74b.

22. Babylonian Talmud, *Shabbat* 128b.

23. *Kitvei Ha-Ramban* [The Writings of Nahmanides], ed. Chaim Chavel (Je-rusalem: Mosad Ha-Rav Kook, 1963), vol. 2, p. 43.

24. See David M. Feldman, *Birth Control in Jewish Law* (New York: New York University Press, 1968; reprinted as *Marital Relations, Birth Control and Abortion in Jewish Law* [New York: Schocken Books, 1974]), pp. 284–94.

25. *Mishneh Torah*, Laws of Ethics, chaps. 1–3.

26. English translations of these works are available. Bachya's *Chovot HaL'vavot* (*Duties of the Heart*) has been translated by Moses Hyamson (New York: Feldheim, 1970); *Sefer HaChinuch* has been translated by Charles Wengrov as *The Book of Mitzvah Education* (New York: Feldheim, 1978–89), 5 vols.; and *Kad HaKemach* has been translated into English by C. Chavel under the title *En-cyclopedia of Torah Thoughts* (New York: Shilo, 1980). Moses Luzzato's *M'silat Y'sharim* has been translated by Mordecai M. Kaplan as *The Path of the Upright* (Philadelphia: Jewish Publication Society, 1936, 1964).

27. *Tosefta, T'rumot* 3:1. One source, though, says that when the intoxication is so great that it amounts to "the drunkenness of Lot" (Genesis 19:33–35)—i.e., to virtual unconsciousness—then such people may be exempt from criminal liabil-ity for what they do in such a state. See Babylonian Talmud, *Eiruvin* 65a.

28. Babylonian Talmud, *N'darim* 22a; *Gittin* 61a. See also Babylonian Talmud, *Avodah Zarah* 55a, where the expression is *l'sayei-a y'dai ovrei aveirah*, "to help those who commit a sin."

Chapter 7: Dementia: Seen by a Neurologist

1. Isaac Bashevis Singer, "Joseph and Koza," in *Stories for Children* (New York: Farrar, Straus and Giroux, 1984), pp. 146–51.

2. Max Vasmer, *Etimologicheskii slovar' russkogo yazyka*, vol. 1 (Moscow: Progress, 1964), p. 99; vol. 4 (Moscow: Progress, 1973), p. 542.

3. Patricia Polacco, *Babushka Baba Yaga* (New York: Philomel, 1993), p. 1.

4. Maurer K, Volk S, and Gerbaldo H. Auguste D and Alzheimer's Disease, *Lancet*, 1997; 349:1546-49.

5. Dr. Alzheimer looked beyond behavior—the face of dementia—to pathology, the biological basis. He was the first to explain what was previously considered a psychiatric disorder in neurological terms. It is still a problem today. For example, insurers still view dementia as a psychiatric condition and insist that neurologists code for psychiatric diagnoses ("senile dementia with or without behavior difficulties") before we give the etiological diagnosis (e.g., Alzheimer's disease, Lewy body disease).

6. Isaac Bashevis Singer, *Stories for Children* (New York: Farrar, Straus and Giroux, 1984), p. 173.

Chapter 8: Doorways of Hope:
Adapting to Alzheimer's

1. Original translation by Sheldon Marder.

2. Robert Davis (with help from his wife, Betty), *My Journey into Alzheimer's Disease* (Carol Stream, IL: Tyndale, 1989), p. 107.

3. Stephen G. Post and Peter J. Whitehouse, "Spirituality, Religion, and Alzheimer's Disease," in *Spiritual Care for Persons with Dementia*, ed. Larry Van de Creek (New York: Haworth Press, 1999), p. 52.

4. The names of residents of the Jewish Home of San Francisco have been changed.

5. David Keck, *Forgetting Whose We Are: Alzheimer's Disease and the Love of God* (Nashville: Abingdon Press, 1996).

6. Moses Maimonides, *Guide of the Perplexed*1:1.

7. Hershel Jonah Matt, "Fading Image of God? Theological Reflections of a Nursing Home Chaplain," *Judaism* 36, no. 1 (Winter 1987): 75–83.

8. Charles Woodman, "Seeking Meaning in Late Stage Dementia," *Journal of Pastoral Care & Counseling* 59, no. 4 (Winter 2005): 335–43.

9. Samuel Dresner, *Prayer, Humility and Compassion* (Philadelphia: Jewish Publication Society, 1957), p. 23.

10. Ted Cohen, "Metaphor and the Cultivation of Intimacy," *Critical Inquiry* 5, no. 1 (Autumn 1978): 3–12.

11. David Mason, "The Inland Sea," in *Beyond Forgetting: Poetry and Prose about Alzheimer's Disease*, ed. Holly J. Hughes (Kent, OH: Kent State University Press, 2009), p. 209.

12. Billy Collins, "Forgetfulness," in *Questions about Angels* (New York: Quill/William Morrow, 1991), pp. 20–21.

13. Donald Capps, "Alzheimer's Disease and the Loss of Self," *Journal of Pastoral Care & Counseling* 62, nos. 1–2 (Spring–Summer 2008): 19–28.

14. Ibid., pp. 25–26.

15. Tess Gallagher, in *Beyond Forgetting*, p. xvii.

16. David Mason, "Home Care," in *Beyond Forgetting*, p. 135.

17. Tess Gallagher, in *Beyond Forgetting*, pp. xix–xx.

18. Rachel, *Flowers of Perhaps*, translated by Robert Friend with Shimon Sandbank. New Milford, CT. The Toby Press, 2008, p. 25.

19. Tess Gallagher, in *Beyond Forgetting*, pp. xvii–xviii.

20. I am indebted to Eileen Shamy, teacher and Methodist clergywoman, who pioneered ministry to people with Alzheimer's disease. I first learned about habilitative care in her book *A Guide to the Spiritual Dimension of Care for People with Alzheimer's Disease and Related Dementia: More than Body, Brain and Breath* (London: Jessica Kingsley Publishers, 2003)—first published in 1997 in New Zealand under the title *More than Body, Brain and Breath*.

Chapter 9: Let There Be Light:
Creative Adaptations to Alzheimer's

1. Rabindranath Tagore, *Heart of God*, ed. Herbert F. Vetter (Boston: Charles E. Tuttle Co., 1997), p. 74.

2. *The Illuminated Rumi*, trans. Coleman Barks (New York: Broadway Books, 1997), p. 2.

Chapter 10: From Frustration to Compassion:
A Neurologist's Perspective

1. Ellen Frankel, *The Classic Tales: 4000 Years of Jewish Lore* (Northvale, NJ: Jason Aronson, 1993).

2. Hayim Nahman Bialik and Yehoshua Hana Ravnitzky, eds., *The Book of Legends*, trans. William G. Braude (New York: Schocken Books, 1992), p. 639, item 274.

3. Ibid., item 275.

4. Ibid., item 276.

5. Roger Rosenblatt, review of *The Boy in the Moon: A Father's Journey to Understand His Extraordinary Son*, by Ian Brown, *New York Times*, May 8, 2011, Sunday Book Review.

Chapter 11: Alzheimer's and the Soul:
A New Perspective

1. Translation from *Mishkan T'filah: A Reform Siddur* (New York: CCAR Press, 2007), p. 32.

2. Ibid., p. 34.

3. It can be found on the CD *As You Go on Your Way: Shacharit—The Morning Prayers*, by Debbie Friedman.

4. *Rabbi's Manual* (New York: CCAR Press, 1988), p. 159, based on Ecclesiastes 12:7.

5. A man offering this prayer would say *Modeh*; a woman offering this prayer would say *Modah*.

6. Translation from *Mishkan T'filah: A Reform Siddur* (New York: CCAR Press, 2007), p. 24.

Chapter 12: Memory Is Incumbent upon the Jew: But What about My Mother's Dementia?

1. *Zakhor: Jewish History and Jewish Memory* (Seattle: University of Washington Press, 1982), p. 5.
2. Soncino edition of the Zohar, Edited and Translated by: Simon, Sperling. Levertoff, NY: Soncino Press, 1996.
3. Barbara Kingsolver, *Animal Dreams*.
4. Yerushalmi, pp. 73–74.
5. Jonathan Safran Foer, *Everything Is Illuminated* (Perennial: Harper Collins, 2003), p. 198.

Chapter 13: Care at Home or Care in a Home?

1. Joseph Telushkin, *The Book of Jewish Values: A Day-by-Day Guide to Ethical Living* (New York: Bell Tower, 2000), p. 347.
2. Ibid.

Chapter 14: He's Still My Father
1. Nancy L. Mace and Peter V. Rabins, *The 36-Hour Day: A Family Guide to Caring for People with Alzheimer Disease, Other Dementias, and Memory Loss in Later Life*, 5th ed. (Baltimore: John Hopkins University Press, 2006).
2. Aviva Gottlieb Zornberg, *Genesis: The Beginning of Desire* (Philadelphia: Jewish Publication Society, 1995), p. 162.
3. Maimonides, *Mishneh Torah*, *Sefer Torah* 10:1. See also CCAR Responsa 5757.4, "Proper Disposal of a Worn *Sefer Torah*," especially notes 4–7.

Chapter 15: The Uncertain Path: Emerging Issues for the Caregiver

1. *Jewish Approaches to Alzheimer's and Dementia*, Bio-ethics Study Guide 15 (New York: Union for Reform Judaism, Department of Jewish Family Concerns, Spring 2009), p. 33.
2. "A Journey with Dementia—the Absence of Presence," Dr. Robert Lester, posted at www.jewishsacredaging.com, Dec 1, 2009.
3. Elliot N. Dorff, *Matters of Life and Death* (Philadelphia: Jewish Publication Society, 1998), p.200.
4. Richard F. Address, "With Eyes Undimmed and Vigor Unabated: Sex, Sexuality, and Older Adults," *CCAR Journal: A Reform Jewish Quarterly*, Fall 2001, p. 64.
5. J. David Bleich, "Can There Be Marriage without Marriage?" *Tradition*, Winter 1999, p. 42.
6. Daniel Schiff, "Separating the Adult from Adultery," in *Marriage and Its Obstacles in Jewish Law*, ed. Walter Jacob and Moshe Zemer (Pittsburgh: Freehof Institute of Progressive Halakhah / Rodef Shalom Press, 1999), p. 80.
7. Phil Bazeley, "Ritual Commemorating Becoming an *Aguneh/Agunah* Due to Illness," Hebrew Union College–Jewish Institute of Religion, 2009.

Chapter 16: The Not-Person

1. Maimonides, *Shemonah Perakim: A Treatise on the Soul*, trans. Leonard S. Kravitz and Kerry M. Olitzky (New York: URJ Press, 1999), pp. 1, 9.
2. *Mishnah Avot* 5:21, in *Mishnayoth*, vol. 4, ed. Philip Blackman (Gateshead, UK: Judaica Press, 1973), pp. 537–38.

Chapter 17: Spiraling Down and Up the Staircase: The Descent of Dementia and the Ascent That Follows

1. See discussion in Stuart Schoffman, "From Heaven to Hypochondria: Metaphors of Jewish Healing," in *Midrash and Medicine: Healing Body and Soul in the Jewish Interpretive Tradition*, ed. William Cutter (Woodstock, VT: Jewish Lights, 2011), pp. 19–26.
2. Ibid., p. 20.
3. Patti Davis, *The Long Goodbye*.
4. The words "in peace" have been added to the JPS translation.

Chapter 18: The Whole World Is Full of God's Glory

1. Stephen G. Post, *The Moral Challenge of Alzheimer's Disease* (Baltimore: Johns Hopkins University Press, 1995), p. 3.
2. Ibid., p. 15, citing Peter Singer in *Practical Ethics* (Cambridge: Cambridge University Press, 1993). To be sure, our culture is not yet at the point where we are prepared to deny caregiving resources to individuals with dementia. But given the current concern about resource availability, we can expect to hear more from those who support such a position. It should also be noted that Dr. Singer, a chief proponent of this school of thought, is the grandson of Holocaust survivors—Jews who were themselves legally categorized by the Nazis as *untermenschen*, "subhuman." The irony I leave to the reader to appreciate.
3. At our facility, we refer to resident "neighborhoods" rather than "nursing units" in order to emphasize and promote a more holistic approach to care.
4. Philip Birnbaum, ed., *Ha-Siddur Ha-Shalem (Daily Prayer Book)* (New York: Hebrew Publishing Co., 1949), p. 74. Cf. Isaiah 6:3.
5. Ibid., p. 332. Cf. also Psalm 115:17, "The dead do not praise God," which certainly could suggest that a living human being, no matter how cognitively compromised, still praises God just by being alive!
6. Maurice Friedman, *Martin Buber: The Life of Dialogue*, 3rd ed. (Chicago: University of Chicago, 1960), p. 85. Cf. also Martin Buber, *The Way of Response* (New York: Schocken Books, 1966), p. 113.
7. Sam Keen, *Fire in the Belly: On Being a Man* (New York: Bantam Books, 1991), p. 170ff.

Permissions

Every attempt has been made to obtain permission to reprint previously published material. The publisher gratefully acknowledges the following for permission to reprint previously published material:

JASON ARONSON PUBLISHERS, INC.: "Hanokh of Alexandria Taught" in *The Classic Tales: 4000 Years of Jewish Lore* edited by Ellen Frankel. Jason Aronson is an imprint of Rowman & Littlefield Publishers, Inc.

ALZHEIMER'S ASSOCIATION: *2011 Alzheimer's Disease Facts and Figures* ©2012 Alzheimer's Association. Printed with permission. All rights reserved.